ISAAC .B. DARLINGTON

CARB CYCLING COOKBOOK FOR WOMEN OVER 50

50+ Delicious Recipes and 14 Days Meal Plan

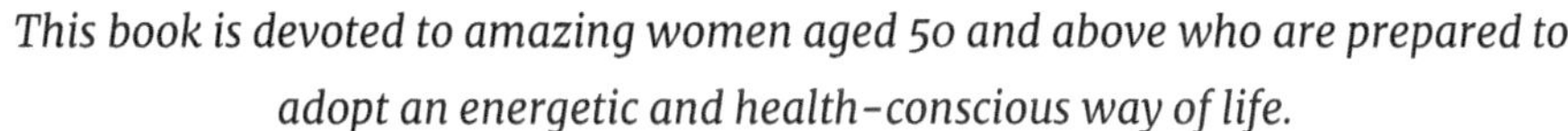

This book is devoted to amazing women aged 50 and above who are prepared to adopt an energetic and health-conscious way of life.

You possess strength, competence, and merit feeling your utmost. This exploration into carb cycling is tailored for you, aiming to reignite your vitality, regulate your weight, and relish flavorful meals throughout the process.

Let's embark on this adventure together, savoring each delightful and nutritious recipe along the way!

Contents

1

Chapter 1

Introduction

My Mother, Agnes (everyone calls her Aggie), turned 66 last year and, like many women her age, started feeling a shift in her energy levels. The walks that used to be effortless now left her winded, and those stairs to her favorite bakery suddenly seemed daunting. She wasn't overweight, but her clothes felt snugger, and the doctor mentioned keeping an eye on her blood sugar. Aggie wasn't one to give up. She'd always been active, volunteering at the local library and taking her dog, Winston, for long walks. But these changes worried her.

One day, while visiting, I saw her flipping through a new book - "Carb Cycling Cookbook for Women Over 50." Intrigued, I asked her about it. Aggie explained how frustrated she was feeling. Dieting seemed restrictive, and she loved her carbs! This book, however, promised a different approach. It talked about giving her body the fuel it craved on certain days, while keeping things balanced. She wasn't just drawn to the delicious recipes, but the idea of feeling strong and in control again.

That week, we started grocery shopping together, picking out colorful vegetables, lean proteins, and whole grains. The kitchen became our happy place, filled with the aroma of new dishes. We laughed over slightly burnt sweet potato toast (practice makes perfect!), and marveled at the vibrant lentil soup. Slowly, Aggie's energy returned. She started walking Winston for longer stretches, even joining a local walking group. Her doctor was impressed with her improved blood sugar levels and overall health.

But do you know what the biggest change was? The twinkle back in Aggie's eyes, she looked more happier than before. Carb cycling wasn't just about food; it was about rediscovering her strength and zest for life. Now, whenever someone asks about her secret, Aggie, with a mischievous grin, pulls out her well-worn cookbook and says, "It's all about the carbs, darling, but the right kind!"

2

Chapter 2

Understanding Carb Cycling: The Why and How for Women Over 50

Carb cycling is a dietary approach alternating between periods of high and low carbohydrate intake, customizable to individual needs and objectives.

Why Carb Cycling Might Be of Interest to Women Over 50

1. Blood Sugar Regulation: Carb cycling can assist in managing blood sugar levels by aligning carbohydrate consumption with activity levels.
2. Boosting Energy: Combatting declining energy levels associated with aging, carb cycling ensures adequate fuel for both physical and cognitive activities.
3. Weight Control: By creating a slight calorie deficit on low-carb days and utilizing carbs for energy on high-carb days, carb cycling aids in weight management.

How Carb Cycling Might Work for Women Over 50

1. Tailoring Carb Intake: Adjusting carb consumption based on daily activity levels, focusing on higher intake on workout days and moderation on rest days.
2. Emphasizing Whole Grains: Prioritizing whole grains as a source of complex carbohydrates for sustained energy and dietary fiber.
3. Monitoring Macronutrients: Tracking carb intake alongside protein and fat ensures a well-rounded diet.

Macronutrient Magic: Carbs, Protein, Fat, and Fiber in Harmony

This section delves into the fascinating realm of macro nutrients! Similar to a magician utilizing various elements to craft illusions, grasping the concepts of macro nutrients - carbohydrates, protein, fat, and fiber - is crucial for orchestrating dietary success for your body, particularly when adhering to a carb cycling regimen.

The Macronutrient Ensemble:

- Carbohydrates: Serving as the primary energy source for our bodies, carbohydrates manifest in both simple and complex forms. While simple carbs offer quick energy but may result in crashes, complex carbs provide sustained energy and dietary fiber.
- Protein: Acting as the fundamental building blocks of our bodies, protein is vital for muscle repair, cellular growth, and hormone balance.
- Fats: Embrace the significance of fats! Healthy fats play pivotal roles in hormone synthesis, cognitive function, and nutrient assimilation.
- Fiber: A staunch ally to our digestive system, fiber facilitates digestion, promotes satiety, and aids in blood sugar regulation.

The Synchronization Principle: Just as a harmonious chord resonates, the magic unfolds when these macronutrients collaborate. Here's how:

- Balanced Meal Composition: Strive for a well-rounded plate at every meal, incorporating complex carbs (such as vegetables and whole grains), lean protein sources, healthy fats (like avocado and nuts), and fiber-rich foods.

- Carb Cycling Synergy: On high-carb days, prioritize complex carbohydrates to fuel your body efficiently. Conversely, on low-carb days, emphasize protein and healthy fats to sustain satiety and energy levels.
- Fiber Enrichment: Integrate fiber-packed foods into your daily meals to promote satiety, regulate digestion, and support stable blood sugar levels.

Guidelines for Macronutrient Equilibrium:

- Mindful Label Reading: Pay attention to the carbohydrate, protein, and fat content listed on food labels. This empowers you to make informed dietary decisions and strategize your meals effectively.
- Meal Planning: Preparing meals ahead of time ensures a diverse array of macronutrients is readily available, minimizing the likelihood of succumbing to unhealthy choices when time is limited.
- Body Awareness: Tune in to your body's responses to various foods. Opt for macronutrient combinations that sustain energy levels and foster satisfaction throughout the day.

By comprehending and synchronizing these macro nutrients, you can curate a personalized carb cycling regimen that optimally fuels your body for enhanced health and vitality beyond the age of 50!

3

Chapter 3

Breakfast Recipes

High-Carb Breakfast Recipes

Berries and Cream Chia Pudding

Ingredients:

- ½ cup chia seeds
- 1 ¼ cups unsweetened almond milk (or your choice of milk)
- ¼ cup fresh or frozen berries (plus extra for garnish)
- 1 tablespoon maple syrup (or your preferred sweetener)
- ½ teaspoon vanilla extract
- Pinch of salt
- ¼ cup sliced almonds or chopped nuts (optional)

Instructions:

1. Combine chia seeds, almond milk, berries, maple syrup, vanilla extract, and salt in a medium bowl, whisking until well blended.

2. Allow the mixture to rest for 5 minutes, enabling the chia seeds to absorb the liquid and swell.
3. Stir the mixture thoroughly. Cover the bowl and refrigerate for at least 3 hours, or overnight for a thicker consistency.
4. When serving, divide the chia pudding into bowls. Garnish with additional fresh berries and sliced almonds or nuts for added crunch and flavor.

Tips:

- To achieve a denser pudding, decrease the almond milk to ¾ cup.
- Store chia pudding in the refrigerator for up to 3 days.
- Feel free to experiment with various milk alternatives, nut varieties, and berry selections.
- Opt for plant-based milk for a vegan-friendly rendition.

Whole-Wheat Pancakes with Nut Butter and Berries

Ingredients:

- 1 cup whole-wheat flour
- 2 teaspoons baking powder
- 1/4 teaspoon baking soda
- 1/4 teaspoon salt
- 1 1/2 cups milk (dairy or non-dairy)
- 1 egg
- 1 tablespoon melted butter or oil
- 1/4 cup mashed banana (optional, for added sweetness)
- 1/4 cup fresh or frozen berries (optional, for batter enhancement)

For Garnish:

- Your preferred nut butter (peanut, almond, cashew, etc.)

- Fresh berries
- Maple syrup (optional)

Instructions:

1. Whisk together whole-wheat flour, baking powder, baking soda, and salt in a large bowl.
2. In another bowl, combine milk, egg, melted butter or oil, and mashed banana (if using).
3. Pour the wet mixture into the dry ingredients and gently stir until just blended. Avoid overmixing; a few lumps are acceptable.
4. If desired, delicately fold fresh or frozen berries into the batter.
5. Heat a lightly greased griddle or pan over medium heat.
6. Pour approximately 1/4 cup of batter for each pancake onto the heated surface.
7. Cook for 2-3 minutes per side, or until golden brown and bubbles form on the surface. Flip the pancakes and cook for an additional 1-2 minutes, or until cooked through.
8. Serve warm pancakes topped with a dollop of your chosen nut butter, fresh berries, and a drizzle of maple syrup (if desired).

Tips:

- Adjust milk quantity for thicker or thinner pancakes.
- Prepare the batter in advance and refrigerate for up to 30 minutes.
- Leftover pancakes can be stored in an airtight container in the refrigerator for up to 2 days and reheated in a microwave or toaster oven.

Scrambled Eggs with Smoked Salmon and Whole-Wheat Toast

Ingredients:

- 2 large eggs

- 1 tablespoon unsweetened almond milk (or your preferred milk)
- Pinch of salt
- Pinch of freshly ground black pepper
- 1 tablespoon butter
- 2 slices whole-wheat bread
- 2 ounces smoked salmon, thinly sliced
- 1 tablespoon chopped fresh chives (optional)

Instructions:

1. In a medium bowl, whisk together eggs, almond milk, salt, and pepper until well combined.
2. Melt butter in a non-stick pan over medium heat. Swirl to coat the pan evenly.
3. Pour in the egg mixture and let it sit briefly. Gently stir the eggs with a rubber spatula, allowing cooked curds to form while pushing the uncooked eggs towards the center.
4. Continue stirring and scraping the pan until the eggs reach your desired consistency, ensuring not to overcook.
5. While the eggs are cooking, toast the whole-wheat bread slices to your preferred level of crispness.
6. Optionally, spread a thin layer of butter on the toasted bread slices.
7. Divide the scrambled eggs evenly between the two toast slices.
8. Top each serving with slices of smoked salmon and sprinkle with chopped chives, if using.
9. Serve immediately and relish the flavors!

Tips:

- For creamier eggs, consider adding a tablespoon of cream cheese or sour cream to the egg mixture before cooking.
- If fresh chives are unavailable, substitute with a pinch of dried chives or another fresh herb of your choice, such as dill.

- To prepare in advance, scramble the eggs and store them in the refrigerator for up to 2 days in an airtight container. Reheat gently in a pan over low heat.

Greek Yogurt Parfait with Granola and Fruit

Ingredients:

- 1 cup plain Greek yogurt (2% fat or higher)
- ¼ cup granola (either homemade or store-bought)
- ½ cup fresh or frozen berries
- ¼ cup chopped nuts (such as almonds, walnuts, or pecans)
- 1 tablespoon honey or maple syrup (optional)
- Mint leaves for garnish (optional)

Instructions:

1. Begin by layering half of the Greek yogurt into a bowl or parfait glass.
2. Sprinkle half of the granola evenly over the yogurt layer.
3. Add half of the berries on top of the granola.
4. Repeat the layering process with the remaining yogurt, granola, and berries.
5. Drizzle the parfait with honey or maple syrup if desired for extra sweetness.
6. Garnish with chopped nuts and a sprig of mint for a decorative touch (optional).

Tips:

- To achieve a thicker yogurt consistency, consider straining the Greek yogurt for about 30 minutes before assembling the parfait.
- Prepare the parfaits ahead of time and store them in airtight containers in the refrigerator overnight. Note that the granola may soften slightly.

- Experiment with various yogurt, granola, fruit, and nut combinations to customize your parfait according to your preferences.
- For a vegan-friendly option, substitute plant-based yogurt for the Greek yogurt.

Vegetable Frittata with Whole-Wheat Toast

Ingredients:

- 1 tablespoon olive oil
- 1 cup chopped vegetables (bell peppers, onions, mushrooms, zucchini, cherry tomatoes - any combination you prefer!)
- 2 cloves garlic, minced
- 6 large eggs
- ¼ cup unsweetened almond milk (or your choice of milk)
- ½ cup shredded low-fat cheese (cheddar, mozzarella, or a blend)
- ¼ cup chopped fresh herbs (optional, such as parsley, basil, or chives)
- Salt and freshly ground black pepper, to taste
- 2 slices whole-wheat bread

Instructions:

1. Preheat your oven to 375°F (190°C). Lightly grease a 10-inch oven-safe skillet or pie dish.
2. Heat olive oil in the skillet over medium heat. Add the chopped vegetables and cook until softened and slightly golden brown, approximately 5-7 minutes. Stir in the minced garlic and cook for an additional minute, until fragrant.
3. In a large bowl, whisk together the eggs and almond milk (or preferred milk). Season generously with salt and pepper. Stir in the shredded cheese and chopped herbs (if using).
4. Pour the egg mixture over the cooked vegetables in the skillet. Gently tilt the pan to ensure even distribution of the eggs and vegetables.

5. Bake the frittata in the preheated oven for 20-25 minutes, or until the center is set and a toothpick inserted comes out clean.
6. While the frittata is baking, toast the whole-wheat bread slices.
7. Once cooked, remove the frittata from the oven and allow it to cool slightly before slicing into wedges.

Tips:

- Get creative with your vegetable choices! This recipe is perfect for using up leftover veggies.
- If you prefer a vegetarian option, simply omit the cheese or substitute it with a vegetarian alternative.
- Leftover frittata wedges can be stored in an airtight container in the refrigerator for up to 3 days. Reheat gently in a pan or microwave for a quick and satisfying breakfast or lunch.

Sweet Potato Toast with Avocado and Eggs

Ingredients:

- 1 large sweet potato
- 1/2 ripe avocado
- 2 large eggs
- 1 tablespoon olive oil, divided
- Pinch of salt and freshly ground black pepper, to taste
- Fresh cilantro or chives, chopped (for garnish)
- Optional: Red pepper flakes for a touch of heat

Instructions:

1. Roast the Sweet Potato: Preheat your oven to 400°F (200°C). Wash and dry the sweet potato. Using a sharp knife, carefully slice the sweet potato into thick rounds (approximately 1/2-inch thick). Toss the slices with 1/2

tablespoon of olive oil, salt, and pepper. Arrange the slices on a baking sheet and roast for 15-20 minutes, or until tender-crisp and golden brown, flipping halfway through.

2. Prepare the Avocado: While the sweet potato roasts, halve, pit, and scoop the avocado flesh into a bowl. Mash the avocado with a fork until creamy. Season with a pinch of salt and pepper (optional: add a squeeze of lemon juice to prevent browning).

3. Cook the Eggs: In a separate pan, heat the remaining 1/2 tablespoon of olive oil over medium heat. Crack the eggs into the pan and cook to your desired doneness (sunny side up, over easy, scrambled). Season with salt and pepper.

4. Assemble & Enjoy: Once the sweet potato slices are cooked, remove them from the oven and arrange them on plates. Spread the mashed avocado evenly over the warm sweet potato toasts. Top each toast with a cooked egg. Garnish with a sprinkle of red pepper flakes (optional) and chopped fresh cilantro or chives.

Tips:

- Short on time? Microwave the sweet potato slices for 4-5 minutes per side on high, flipping halfway through, until tender. However, oven-roasting provides a crispier texture.
- For a creamier avocado spread, consider mixing it with a tablespoon of plain Greek yogurt or ricotta cheese.
- Feel free to personalize with additional toppings such as crumbled feta cheese, a drizzle of balsamic glaze, or a sprinkle of everything bagel seasoning.

Oatmeal with Nuts, Seeds, and Fruit

Ingredients:

- 1/2 cup rolled oats (old-fashioned or quick oats)

- 1 cup unsweetened almond milk (or your preferred milk)
- 1/4 cup water
- Pinch of salt
- 1/4 cup chopped nuts (such as almonds, walnuts, or pecans)
- 2 tablespoons chia seeds or flaxseeds
- 1/4 cup fresh or frozen berries
- 1 tablespoon honey or maple syrup (optional)

Instructions:

1. In a medium saucepan, combine the rolled oats, almond milk, water, and salt. Bring the mixture to a boil over medium heat, stirring occasionally.
2. Once boiling, reduce the heat to low and simmer for 3-5 minutes, or until the oats reach your desired consistency (creamy or with a bit more bite).
3. While the oatmeal simmers, toast the chopped nuts in a dry skillet over medium heat for a few minutes until fragrant and lightly golden brown. Be careful not to burn them.
4. Remove the oatmeal from the heat and spoon it into a bowl.
5. Top the oatmeal with the toasted nuts, chia seeds or flaxseeds, and fresh or frozen berries.
6. Drizzle with honey or maple syrup for additional sweetness if desired (optional).

Breakfast Burrito Bowl with Whole-Wheat Tortilla

Ingredients:

i. Scrambled Eggs:

- 2 large eggs
- 1 tablespoon unsweetened almond milk (or your preferred milk)
- Pinch of salt
- Pinch of freshly ground black pepper

- 1 tablespoon olive oil

ii. Breakfast Bowl:

- ½ cup cooked black beans (rinsed and drained)
- ½ cup chopped vegetables (such as bell peppers, onions, mushrooms, spinach)
- ¼ cup shredded cheese (cheddar, Monterey Jack, or a blend)
- ¼ cup chopped fresh salsa (optional)
- 1 avocado, sliced or mashed
- 1 whole-wheat tortilla, warmed
- Fresh cilantro or chives, chopped (for garnish)
- Hot sauce (optional)

Instructions:

1. Prepare the Scrambled Eggs: In a medium bowl, whisk together the eggs, almond milk, salt, and pepper.
2. Heat olive oil in a non-stick pan over medium heat. Once hot, pour in the egg mixture and cook, stirring constantly with a rubber spatula, until the eggs are scrambled to your desired consistency (soft scrambled or slightly firmer). Set aside.
3. Assemble the Bowl: In a large bowl, combine the cooked black beans, chopped vegetables, and shredded cheese.
4. Top with the scrambled eggs, salsa (if using), sliced or mashed avocado, and a sprinkle of chopped fresh cilantro or chives.
5. Warm up the whole-wheat tortilla in a dry skillet or microwave for a few seconds.
6. Serve the breakfast bowl with the warmed whole-wheat tortilla on the side, allowing you to scoop up the ingredients and enjoy it burrito-style or mix everything together in the bowl.
7. Add a drizzle of hot sauce for an extra kick if desired (optional).

Smoothie with Protein Powder, Greens, and Fruit

Ingredients:

- 1 cup unsweetened almond milk (or your preferred milk)
- 1 scoop protein powder (such as chocolate, vanilla, or your favorite flavor)
- ½ cup frozen spinach or kale
- ½ cup fresh or frozen berries (blueberries, raspberries, strawberries)
- ½ banana
- ¼ cup chopped avocado (optional, for extra creaminess)
- 1 tablespoon chia seeds (optional, for added fiber)
- 1 tablespoon honey or maple syrup (optional, for additional sweetness)

Instructions:

1. Combine all ingredients (almond milk, protein powder, spinach or kale, berries, banana, avocado if using, chia seeds if using, and honey or maple syrup if using) in a blender.
2. Blend on high speed until smooth and creamy. If the smoothie is too thick, add a bit more almond milk or water to reach your desired consistency.
3. Pour the smoothie into a glass and enjoy its goodness!

Tips:

- Experiment with different types of protein powder, greens, fruits, and milk to create your preferred flavor combinations.
- To thicken the smoothie, opt for frozen fruit instead of fresh.
- If fresh spinach or kale isn't available, use a handful of baby spinach or a scoop of greens powder.
- Prepare this smoothie in advance by blending all ingredients except the protein powder. Store the mixture in the freezer in an airtight container for up to 2 days. When ready to enjoy, blend it again with the protein powder.

Whole-Wheat French Toast with Berries and Maple Syrup

Ingredients:

- 2 large eggs
- 1/2 cup unsweetened almond milk (or your preferred milk)
- 1/4 cup water
- 1 teaspoon vanilla extract
- 1/4 teaspoon ground cinnamon
- Pinch of salt
- 4 slices whole-wheat bread
- 1 tablespoon butter
- 1 cup fresh berries (blueberries, raspberries, strawberries)
- Maple syrup, to taste

Instructions:

1. In a shallow dish, whisk together eggs, almond milk, water, vanilla extract, cinnamon, and salt until thoroughly combined.
2. Heat a large skillet or griddle over medium heat and melt the butter in the pan.
3. Dip each slice of whole-wheat bread into the egg mixture, ensuring it's soaked on both sides.
4. Transfer the soaked bread slices to the preheated skillet and cook for 2-3 minutes per side until they turn golden brown and are cooked through.
5. While the french toast cooks, prepare the berries by washing them gently and slicing them if desired.
6. Once cooked, place the french toast slices on a plate.
7. Top each slice generously with fresh berries.
8. Drizzle maple syrup over the french toast according to your taste.

Tips:

- Opt for thicker slices of whole-wheat bread for a heartier french toast experience.
- If the egg mixture seems too thin, you can add a tablespoon of flour to slightly thicken it.
- For a richer flavor, substitute some of the almond milk with heavy cream or half-and-half.
- This recipe can easily be scaled up to serve more people if needed.

Low-Carb Breakfast Recipes (for Feeling Fulfilled)

Eggs with Wilted Greens and Smoked Salmon

Ingredients:

- 2 large eggs
- 1 tablespoon olive oil
- 2-3 cups leafy greens (spinach, arugula, kale - any mix you prefer!)
- 1 clove garlic, minced (optional)
- Salt and freshly ground black pepper, to taste
- 2 ounces smoked salmon, thinly sliced
- 1 tablespoon chopped fresh chives (optional)
- 1 tablespoon hemp seeds (optional)

Instructions:

1: Prepare the Eggs: Select your preferred egg-cooking method:

- For fried eggs: Heat a pan with olive oil over medium heat. Crack eggs into the pan and cook to your liking (sunny side up, over easy, or fried).
- For poached eggs: Poach eggs in simmering water with a splash of vinegar until whites are set and yolks are runny.
- For scrambled eggs: Whisk eggs with water, then scramble in a pan with olive oil until cooked through.

2: Wilted Greens: While eggs cook, heat olive oil in a skillet over medium heat. Add greens (and minced garlic, if desired) and sauté until wilted and softened. Season with salt and pepper.

3: Assemble the Dish: Divide wilted greens onto plates. Top each with smoked salmon slices and a cooked egg.

4: Garnish with chopped fresh chives (optional) and hemp seeds (optional) for added healthy fats and nutty flavor.

Tips:

- Experiment with various leafy greens and herbs for diverse flavors.
- For creaminess, add a spoonful of cream cheese or ricotta cheese to wilted greens after softening.
- Store leftover wilted greens in the fridge in an airtight container for up to a day.

Avocado Omelet with Cheese and Peppers

Ingredients:

- 3 large eggs
- 1 tablespoon olive oil
- ¼ cup chopped bell peppers (choose any combination of colors you prefer!)
- ¼ cup chopped red onion (optional)
- 1/4 cup shredded cheese (cheddar, Monterey Jack, or a mix)
- 1/2 ripe avocado, sliced
- Salt and freshly ground black pepper, to taste
- Fresh herbs (optional, like parsley, chives, or cilantro) for garnish

Instructions:

1. Prepare the Eggs: Whisk the eggs in a medium bowl with a pinch of salt and pepper.
2. Sauté the Vegetables: Heat olive oil in a non-stick skillet over medium heat. Add chopped bell peppers (and red onion, if using) and cook for 2-3 minutes until softened. Season with salt and pepper.
3. Cook the Omelet: Pour whisked eggs into the skillet with the vegetables. Tilt the pan to spread the eggs evenly and cook for 1-2 minutes until the edges start setting.
4. Assemble the Omelet: Sprinkle half of the shredded cheese over one side of the omelet and top with sliced avocado.
5. Once the bottom of the omelet is cooked through and the edges are set, carefully fold it in half with a spatula.
6. Cook for another 1-2 minutes until the cheese is melted and the omelet is cooked to your preference.
7. Slide the omelet onto a plate and garnish with the remaining shredded cheese and fresh herbs if desired.

Tips:

- Experiment with different cheeses and veggies. For a vegetarian version, skip the cheese.
- Avoid overcooking the eggs for a fluffy omelet.
- Store any leftovers in the fridge in an airtight container for up to 1 day and reheat gently before serving.

Chia Pudding with Nut Butter and MCT Oil

Ingredients:

- ½ cup unsweetened almond milk (or your preferred milk)
- ¼ cup chia seeds
- 2 tablespoons unsweetened nut butter (almond, peanut, cashew - pick your favorite)

- 1 tablespoon MCT oil
- 1 teaspoon sweetener (optional, like stevia, erythritol, or monk fruit)
- Pinch of salt
- ¼ cup chopped nuts and berries (for topping)

Instructions:

1. Whisk together almond milk, chia seeds, nut butter, MCT oil, optional sweetener, and salt in a small bowl or jar until thoroughly combined.
2. Cover the bowl or jar tightly and refrigerate for at least 4 hours, preferably overnight, to allow the chia seeds to absorb the liquid and create a thick pudding consistency.
3. After chilling, give the pudding a good stir before serving.
4. Divide the chia pudding into two serving bowls.
5. Sprinkle your favorite chopped nuts and berries on top for added crunch and flavor.

Tips:

- Experiment with different nut butter and milk varieties to vary the flavor profile.
- For added creaminess, consider incorporating a tablespoon of full-fat coconut milk or heavy cream (which slightly increases carb content).
- This pudding can be prepared in advance. Make it the night before and store it in the refrigerator for up to 5 days.

Breakfast Sausage with Scramble Eggs

Ingredients:

- 4 ounces breakfast sausage (opt for a low-carb variety)
- 1 tablespoon olive oil
- 2 large eggs

- 1/4 cup diced bell peppers (choose your preferred colors)
- 1/4 cup diced onion (optional)
- Salt and pepper, to taste
- 1/4 cup shredded cheese (cheddar, Monterey Jack, or a blend - optional)
- Fresh herbs, chopped (optional, such as parsley, chives, or cilantro) for garnish

Instructions:

1. Cook the Sausage: Heat olive oil in a large skillet over medium heat. Add the breakfast sausage and cook until browned and fully cooked, breaking it apart with a spatula as needed. Drain any excess fat from the pan.
2. Sauté the Vegetables (Optional): If desired, add the diced bell peppers (and onion, if using) to the skillet with the cooked sausage. Sauté until tender, seasoning with salt and pepper.
3. Prepare the Eggs: In a separate bowl, whisk together the eggs with a splash of water or milk, along with a pinch of salt and pepper.
4. Scramble the Eggs: Push the sausage and vegetables (if using) to one side of the skillet. If necessary, add a bit more olive oil to the empty side. Pour in the whisked eggs and scramble until cooked to your preferred consistency.
5. Combine Ingredients: Once the eggs are cooked, mix them with the sausage and vegetables in the skillet.
6. Add Cheese (Optional): Stir in the shredded cheese, if desired, and heat until melted.
7. Serve: Transfer the dish to plates and garnish with chopped fresh herbs, if using.

Tips:

- Opt for breakfast sausage labeled as "low-carb" or with a higher meat content.
- Feel free to experiment with different veggies, such as mushrooms or

spinach.

- To enhance creaminess, consider incorporating cream cheese or ricotta after cooking the eggs.
- Leftovers can be refrigerated in an airtight container for up to a day and reheated as needed.

Smoked Salmon Cream Cheese on Cucumber Slices

Ingredients:

- 1 large English cucumber, thinly sliced (approximately 20 slices)
- 4 ounces thinly sliced smoked salmon
- 4 ounces softened cream cheese
- 1 tablespoon chopped fresh chives or dill (optional)
- Freshly ground black pepper, to taste

Instructions:

1. Prep the Cucumbers: Rinse and pat dry the English cucumber. Slice it thinly into rounds, about 1/4-inch thick, and arrange them on a serving platter.
2. Prepare the Cream Cheese Spread: Mix the softened cream cheese with freshly ground black pepper in a small bowl. Optionally, incorporate chopped fresh chives or dill for enhanced flavor.
3. Assemble the Appetizers: Spread a thin layer of the cream cheese mixture onto each cucumber slice.
4. Add the Smoked Salmon: Place a piece of smoked salmon atop each cream cheese-covered cucumber slice.
5. Serve Immediately: Indulge in this refreshing and flavorful breakfast offering promptly.

Tips:

- For a smoother spread, blend a tablespoon of sour cream or plain Greek yogurt with the cream cheese.
- Experiment with various herbs, such as parsley or tarragon, as alternatives to chives or dill.
- To streamline preparation, opt for pre-sliced cucumber rounds.
- Leftover cream cheese spread can be refrigerated in an airtight container for up to three days, though it's best to assemble the dish with fresh cucumber slices for optimal texture.

Keto Waffles with Almond Flour and Berries

Ingredients:

- 1 cup almond flour
- 3 large eggs
- 1/4 cup unsweetened almond milk (or your preferred milk)
- 2 tablespoons melted butter or coconut oil
- 2 teaspoons baking powder
- 1/4 teaspoon salt
- 1/4 teaspoon ground cinnamon (optional)
- 1/4 cup fresh or frozen berries (optional)
- Sugar-free maple syrup or erythritol sweetener, to taste (optional)

Instructions:

1. Preheat Waffle Iron: Heat your waffle iron as per the manufacturer's instructions.
2. Blend Dry Ingredients: Combine almond flour, baking powder, and cinnamon (if desired) in a medium bowl, whisking them together.
3. Mix Wet Ingredients: In another bowl, blend eggs, almond milk, melted butter or coconut oil, and salt until thoroughly incorporated.
4. Blend Wet & Dry Ingredients: Gently fold the wet ingredients into the dry mixture until just combined, avoiding overmixing. If using berries,

delicately fold them into the batter.

5. Cook the Waffles: Pour the batter evenly onto the preheated waffle iron. Adjust the batter quantity based on your waffle iron's size. Cook according to the appliance's instructions, or until the waffles turn golden brown and cook through (typically around 3-5 minutes).

6. Serve Warm: Present the waffles hot, optionally drizzled with sugar-free maple syrup or erythritol sweetener, and adorned with fresh berries if not already incorporated into the batter.

Tips:

- Allow the batter to rest briefly before cooking to enhance the waffles' fluffiness by allowing the almond flour to absorb moisture.
- Opt for melted coconut oil for crisper waffles.
- Explore diverse extracts or spices, such as almond extract or nutmeg, to introduce various flavors.
- Refrigerate any leftover waffles in an airtight container for up to 2 days, reheating them gently in a toaster or microwave.

Protein Pancakes with Almond Flour and Berries

Ingredients:

- 1 cup almond flour
- 1 scoop unflavored or vanilla protein powder
- 1/2 teaspoon baking powder
- 1/4 teaspoon salt
- 1 cup unsweetened almond milk (or your preferred milk)
- 2 large eggs
- 1/4 teaspoon vanilla extract (optional)
- 1/2 cup fresh or frozen berries (such as blueberries, raspberries, or mixed berries)
- Sugar-free maple syrup or erythritol sweetener, to taste (optional)

- Butter or coconut oil for cooking

Instructions:

1. Blend Dry Ingredients: In a medium bowl, whisk together almond flour, protein powder, baking powder, and salt.
2. Mix Wet Ingredients: In a separate bowl, whisk almond milk, eggs, and vanilla extract (if using) until thoroughly blended.
3. Combine Wet & Dry Ingredients: Pour the wet mixture into the dry mixture and gently fold with a spatula until just combined. Avoid overmixing. Carefully fold in the berries.
4. Heat Pan: Heat a lightly greased non-stick pan or griddle over medium heat. Melt a small amount of butter or coconut oil in the pan.
5. Cook the Pancakes: Pour about 1/4 cup of batter per pancake onto the preheated pan. Cook for 2–3 minutes per side, or until golden brown and cooked through. Look for bubbles on the pancake surface as an indication to flip.
6. Serve Warm: Serve the pancakes hot, optionally drizzled with sugar-free maple syrup or erythritol sweetener, and topped with additional fresh berries if desired.

Tips:

- Let the batter rest for 5 minutes before cooking to allow the almond flour to absorb moisture and create fluffier pancakes.
- Adjust batter thickness by adding a tablespoon or two of almond milk until reaching a pourable consistency.
- Avoid overcooking pancakes, as they will continue cooking slightly off the heat.
- Store leftover pancakes in an airtight container in the refrigerator for up to 2 days. Reheat gently in a toaster or microwave.

Hard-Boiled Eggs with Sliced Tomatoes and Avocado

Ingredients:

- 2 large hard-boiled eggs
- 1 medium tomato, sliced
- 1/2 ripe avocado, sliced
- Extra virgin olive oil, for drizzling
- Salt and freshly ground black pepper, to taste

Optional additions:

- Chopped fresh herbs (like parsley, chives, or cilantro)
- Your preferred cheese (such as feta or crumbled blue cheese)
- A drizzle of balsamic vinegar glaze

Instructions:

1. Prepare the Eggs: Cook the hard-boiled eggs using your preferred method, such as boiling them for 10-12 minutes and then peeling them under cool running water.
2. Assemble the Dish: Arrange the sliced tomatoes on a plate, followed by the sliced avocado and peeled hard-boiled eggs.
3. Seasoning: Drizzle with olive oil and season with salt and pepper to taste.
4. Optional Additions: Enhance the dish with chopped fresh herbs, a sprinkle of cheese, or a drizzle of balsamic vinegar glaze for extra flavor.

Tips:

- Save time by purchasing pre-cooked hard-boiled eggs.
- Prevent avocado browning by immediately squeezing fresh lemon juice over it.
- Pair this dish with low-carb greens like spinach or arugula for a heartier

breakfast.

Greek Yogurt with Chia Seeds and Berries

Ingredients:

- 1 cup plain full-fat Greek yogurt
- ¼ cup chia seeds
- ¼ cup unsweetened almond milk (or your preferred milk)
- ½ cup fresh or frozen berries (such as blueberries, raspberries, or a mix)
- Sweetener (optional, like stevia, erythritol, or monk fruit)
- ¼ cup chopped nuts (like almonds, walnuts, or pecans - optional)
- Fresh mint leaves (optional, for garnish)

Instructions:

1. Prepare Chia Seed Pudding: Mix 2 tablespoons of chia seeds with 2 tablespoons of almond milk in a small bowl or jar. Let it sit for at least 15 minutes until the chia seeds thicken.
2. Layer the Parfait: Start with half of the Greek yogurt in a serving glass or bowl, followed by half of the berries.
3. Add Chia Seed Layer: Spoon the prepared chia seed pudding over the berries.
4. Complete the Layers: Add the remaining Greek yogurt and top with the remaining berries.
5. Optional Sweetness: Drizzle a bit of sweetener over the top layer if desired.
6. Optional Garnish: Sprinkle chopped nuts over the top and garnish with fresh mint leaves for an attractive presentation.

Tips:

- Prepare the chia seed pudding ahead and store it in the refrigerator for up to 2 days.

- Experiment with different yogurt flavors like vanilla for added sweetness.
- Opt for whole milk yogurt for a creamier texture (slightly higher carb count).
- Leftover parfait can be refrigerated for up to 2 days, though the texture may change slightly.

Additional Low-Carb Variations:

- Spice it Up: Enhance the Greek yogurt with a pinch of cinnamon, nutmeg, or ginger.
- Chocolate Twist: Mix in unsweetened cocoa powder for a chocolatey version (slightly higher carb count).
- Coconut Cream Variation: Substitute half the Greek yogurt with unsweetened coconut yogurt for a tropical flavor.

Frittata Cups with Vegetables and Cheese

Ingredients:

- 6 large eggs
- ¼ cup unsweetened almond milk (or your preferred milk)
- ½ cup chopped veggies (bell peppers, onions, mushrooms, broccoli, spinach)
- ¼ cup shredded cheese (cheddar, Monterey Jack, or a mix)
- Salt and pepper to taste

Optional additions:

- Cooked breakfast sausage or chicken for added protein
- Fresh herbs (parsley, chives, cilantro)
- Low-carb chopped nuts (almonds, walnuts)

Instructions:

1. Preheat Oven: Heat your oven to 375°F (190°C). Grease a muffin tin with cooking spray or olive oil.
2. Whisk Eggs: In a bowl, whisk together eggs and almond milk. Season with salt and pepper.
3. Prepare Vegetables (Optional): If using raw veggies, sauté them in a skillet until soft, then let cool before adding to the egg mixture.
4. Mix Ingredients: Combine veggies (and cooked protein, if using) with the egg mixture. Add cheese and any other desired additions.
5. Fill Muffin Tin: Divide the mixture evenly among muffin cups.
6. Bake: Bake for 18-20 minutes until set and golden brown. Test doneness with a toothpick.
7. Cool and Serve: Allow frittatas to cool slightly before removing from the tin. Serve warm or at room temperature.

Tips:

- Experiment with different veggie and cheese combinations.
- Use leftover cooked veggies for a quick breakfast.
- Store leftovers in the fridge for up to 3 days. Reheat before serving.

Chapter 4

Lunch Recipes

High-Carb Lunch Options

Quinoa Salad with Roasted Vegetables and Chickpeas

Ingredients:

- 1 cup uncooked quinoa, rinsed
- 1 ½ cups vegetable broth
- 2 cups chopped veggies (bell peppers, onions, zucchini, broccoli, cherry tomatoes)
- 1 (15 oz) can chickpeas, drained and rinsed
- 1 tablespoon olive oil
- 1 tablespoon balsamic vinegar
- ½ teaspoon dried oregano
- Salt and pepper to taste

Optional additions:

- ¼ cup crumbled feta cheese
- ¼ cup chopped fresh herbs (parsley, cilantro, mint)
- Cooked chicken or grilled shrimp for extra protein
- Your favorite vinaigrette dressing

Instructions:

1. Cook Quinoa: Combine rinsed quinoa and vegetable broth in a saucepan. Bring to a boil, then simmer, covered, for 15-20 minutes until fluffy. Set aside to cool slightly.
2. Roast Vegetables: Preheat oven to 400°F (200°C). Toss veggies with olive oil, salt, and pepper. Roast on a lined baking sheet for 15-20 minutes until tender and golden.
3. Prepare Dressing: Whisk balsamic vinegar, olive oil, and oregano in a small bowl. Season with salt and pepper.
4. Assemble Salad: In a large bowl, mix cooked quinoa, roasted veggies, and chickpeas. Pour dressing over and toss to coat.
5. Serve: Enjoy salad at room temperature or chilled.

Tips:

- Experiment with different veggie combinations, including root veggies for variety.
- Marinate chickpeas in olive oil and spices before roasting for extra flavor.
- Use leftover roasted veggies in other dishes.
- Store leftovers in the fridge for up to 3 days, refreshing with extra dressing if needed.

Turkey and Avocado Wrap on Whole-Wheat Tortilla

Ingredients:

- 1 large whole-wheat tortilla

- 3-4 ounces thinly sliced deli turkey breast
- 1/2 ripe avocado, sliced
- 2 tablespoons hummus (optional)
- 1-2 tablespoons plain Greek yogurt (optional)
- 1 tomato, sliced
- ¼ cup chopped lettuce or spinach
- Salt and freshly ground black pepper, to taste

Optional additions:

- Chopped cucumber or bell peppers
- A sprinkle of shredded cheese
- A drizzle of your favorite dressing (vinaigrette, ranch)

Instructions:

1. Warm Tortilla (Optional): Heat tortilla in a skillet or microwave until soft and pliable.
2. Spread (Optional): Spread hummus or Greek yogurt on the tortilla.
3. Layer Ingredients: Place turkey, avocado, tomato, and lettuce/spinach on the tortilla. Season with salt and pepper.
4. Add Extras (Optional): Include any additional ingredients like cucumber, bell peppers, or cheese.
5. Roll and Enjoy: Roll the tortilla tightly, starting from the bottom.
6. Serve: Cut the wrap in half and serve immediately.

Tips:

- Choose a soft, high-quality whole-wheat tortilla.
- Prevent avocado browning by drizzling with lemon juice.
- Store leftovers in the fridge for up to 1 day.

Lentil Soup with Whole-Grain Bread

Ingredients:

- 1 tablespoon olive oil
- 1 medium onion, chopped
- 2 carrots, chopped
- 2 celery stalks, chopped
- 2 cloves garlic, minced
- 1 teaspoon dried thyme
- 1 teaspoon ground cumin
- 1/2 teaspoon dried oregano
- 1 cup brown lentils, rinsed
- 4 cups vegetable broth
- 1 (14.5 oz) can diced tomatoes, undrained
- 4 cups chopped kale or spinach
- Slices of whole-grain bread for serving
- Salt and freshly ground black pepper, to taste

Optional additions:

- 1 bay leaf
- 1 tablespoon tomato paste
- A sprinkle of red pepper flakes for a touch of heat

Instructions:

1. Sauté the Vegetables: Heat olive oil in a large pot over medium heat. Add onions, carrots, and celery. Sauté until softened, about 5-7 minutes.
2. Add Spices and Garlic: Stir in minced garlic, thyme, cumin, and oregano. Cook for another minute to release the fragrance.
3. Cook Lentils: Add lentils and vegetable broth to the pot. Bring to a boil, then reduce heat and simmer for 20-25 minutes until lentils are tender.

4. Add Tomatoes and Greens: Mix in diced tomatoes and chopped kale/spinach. Simmer for an additional 5 minutes until greens are wilted.

5. Seasoning: Season with salt and pepper to taste. Optionally, add a bay leaf for extra flavor.

6. Serve: Ladle soup into bowls and serve hot with slices of whole-grain bread.

Tips:

- Experiment with different veggies or use frozen ones.
- For thicker soup, mash some cooked lentils.
- Store leftovers in the fridge for up to 3 days.

Black Bean Burgers on Whole-Wheat Buns

Ingredients:

- 1 (15 oz) can black beans, rinsed and drained
- ½ cup cooked brown rice (optional, for added texture)
- ½ cup rolled oats
- 1 small onion, chopped
- 1 red bell pepper, chopped (optional)
- 2 cloves garlic, minced
- 1 tablespoon olive oil
- 1 egg, lightly beaten
- ½ cup chopped fresh cilantro
- 1 tablespoon chili powder
- 1 teaspoon cumin
- ½ teaspoon dried oregano
- Salt and freshly ground black pepper, to taste
- Hamburger buns (whole-wheat recommended)
- Toppings of your choice (lettuce, tomato, onion, avocado, cheese, salsa,

guacamole)

Instructions:

1. Mash the Beans: Mash about half of the black beans in a large bowl, leaving the other half slightly chunky for texture.
2. Sauté the Vegetables (Optional): Heat olive oil in a skillet over medium heat. Sauté chopped onion and red bell pepper (if using) for 5-7 minutes until softened. Add minced garlic and cook for another minute.
3. Combine Ingredients: In the bowl with mashed beans, add cooked brown rice (if using), rolled oats, cooked vegetables (if using), egg, chopped cilantro, chili powder, cumin, oregano, salt, and pepper. Mix thoroughly.
4. Form the Patties: Shape the bean mixture into 4 patties.
5. Cook the Burgers: Heat a lightly oiled skillet or grill pan over medium heat. Cook the burgers for 4-5 minutes per side until browned and heated through.
6. Toast the Buns (Optional): Lightly toast the hamburger buns in a toaster or skillet for added texture (optional).
7. Assemble and Serve: Place cooked burger patties on the toasted buns, add desired toppings, and enjoy!

Tips:

- Add breadcrumbs if the mixture seems too wet to help bind the ingredients.
- Experiment with various toppings, cheeses, vegetables, and sauces for different flavor combinations.
- Store leftover cooked burgers in an airtight container in the refrigerator for up to 3 days and reheat gently before serving.

Salmon with Brown Rice and Roasted Asparagus

Ingredients:

- 2 (6-ounce) salmon fillets
- 1 tablespoon olive oil
- Salt and freshly ground black pepper, to taste
- 1 cup uncooked brown rice
- 1 ½ cups vegetable broth
- 1 bunch asparagus, trimmed
- 1 tablespoon balsamic vinegar (optional)
- 1 tablespoon chopped fresh parsley (optional, for garnish)

Instructions:

1: Marinate the Salmon (Optional): Combine 1 tablespoon of olive oil with salt and pepper in a shallow dish. Coat the salmon fillets evenly with the marinade and let them marinate for 15 minutes at room temperature for added flavor (optional).

2: Cook the Brown Rice: Simmer uncooked brown rice with vegetable broth in a saucepan for 45-50 minutes until fluffy and fully cooked.

3: Preheat Oven (Optional): Preheat the grill to medium-high heat for grilling or preheat the oven to 400°F (200°C) for baking.

4: Roast the Asparagus: Toss trimmed asparagus with olive oil, salt, and pepper. Roast on a baking sheet for 10-15 minutes until tender-crisp and lightly browned.

5: Cook the Salmon:

i. For grilling: Oil the grill grates and grill the salmon fillets for 4-5 minutes per side until cooked through and slightly flaky.

ii. For baking: Bake the salmon on a parchment-lined baking sheet for 12–15 minutes until cooked through and slightly flaky.

6: Assemble and Serve: Flake the cooked salmon onto plates. Serve with cooked brown rice and roasted asparagus. Optionally, drizzle with balsamic vinegar and garnish with fresh parsley.

Tips:

- Opt for thick-cut salmon fillets for even cooking.
- Test the salmon's doneness by gently pressing the center; if it flakes easily and feels slightly firm, it's ready.
- Store leftover salmon and rice in an airtight container in the fridge for up to 3 days. Reheat gently before serving. Enjoy the roasted asparagus fresh.

Additional Variations:

- Lemon Herb Infusion: Squeeze fresh lemon juice over the cooked salmon and garnish with dill or chives for a zesty twist.
- Asian-Inspired Glaze: Create a glaze with soy sauce, honey, and ginger; brush it onto the salmon during the last few minutes of cooking for an Asian flair.
- Spicy Accent: Drizzle sriracha or your preferred hot sauce over the cooked salmon for a fiery kick.

Chicken Stir-Fry with Whole-Wheat Noodles and Vegetables

Ingredients:

- 1 pound thinly sliced boneless, skinless chicken breasts or thighs
- 1 tablespoon cornstarch

- 2 tablespoons soy sauce
- 1 tablespoon rice vinegar
- 1 tablespoon vegetable oil
- 2 cloves minced garlic
- 1 small sliced onion
- 1 sliced red bell pepper
- 1 cup broccoli florets
- ½ cup sugar snap peas (or snow peas)
- 8 ounces whole-wheat noodles, cooked per package instructions
- Salt and freshly ground black pepper, to taste

Optional additions:

- Chopped carrots or baby corn
- Sesame seeds for garnish
- Chopped fresh cilantro or green onions for garnish
- 1 scrambled egg (for added protein)

Instructions:

1. Marinate the Chicken: In a bowl, mix the sliced chicken with cornstarch, soy sauce, and rice vinegar. Let it marinate for 15-30 minutes.
2. Cook the Noodles: Cook the whole-wheat noodles according to package instructions. Rinse under cold water and set aside.
3. Prepare the Vegetables: Wash and chop the vegetables (onion, bell pepper, broccoli, sugar snap peas).
4. Heat the Pan: Heat vegetable oil in a large skillet or wok over high heat.
5. Cook the Chicken: Add the marinated chicken to the hot pan and stir-fry until cooked through and golden brown, about 4-5 minutes. Remove and set aside.
6. Sauté the Vegetables: In the same pan, add garlic and onion, sauté for 30 seconds. Then add bell pepper, broccoli, and sugar snap peas, stir-fry for 3-4 minutes until tender-crisp.

7. Combine and Season: Return cooked chicken to the pan along with cooked noodles. Season with salt and pepper, toss to combine and heat through.
8. Serve: Divide the stir-fry onto plates. Garnish with sesame seeds, cilantro, or green onions if desired.

Tips:

- Use a large skillet or wok for even cooking.
- Add water or chicken broth if the pan seems dry while stir-frying.
- Experiment with different vegetables.

Tuna Salad Sandwich on Whole-Wheat Bread

Ingredients:

- 2 slices whole-wheat bread (optional: toasted)
- 5 oz canned tuna in water, drained
- 2 tablespoons mayonnaise (or light mayonnaise)
- 1 tablespoon chopped celery
- ½ cup chopped red onion (optional, for added bite)
- ¼ cup chopped fresh parsley
- Salt and freshly ground black pepper, to taste

Optional additions:

- ¼ cup chopped grapes or dried cranberries (for sweetness)
- 1 tablespoon chopped walnuts or pecans (for crunch)
- Shredded cheese
- Lettuce or spinach leaves

Instructions:

1. Prepare the Tuna: Flake the drained tuna with a fork in a medium bowl.

2. Mix the Filling: Combine flaked tuna, mayonnaise, chopped celery, red onion (if using), and chopped parsley. Season with salt and pepper. Mix well.

3. Toast the Bread (Optional): Toast whole-wheat bread slices for a crispier texture if desired.

4. Assemble the Sandwich: Spread tuna salad mixture evenly on one slice of bread. Add optional ingredients like grapes, nuts, cheese, or lettuce/spinach. Top with the other bread slice.

5. Serve: Cut the sandwich in half, diagonally if preferred, and enjoy!

Tips:

- Adjust mayonnaise or add Greek yogurt for a creamier consistency.
- For chunkier tuna salad, flake the tuna less.
- Store leftover tuna salad in the refrigerator for up to 2 days. Serve on crackers or lettuce leaves for a lighter meal.

Vegetarian Chili with Cornbread

Ingredients:

i. For the Chili:

- 1 tbsp olive oil
- 1 medium onion, finely chopped
- 2 cloves garlic, minced
- 1 green bell pepper, finely diced
- 1 (15 oz) can diced tomatoes, not drained
- 1 (15 oz) can black beans, rinsed and drained
- 1 (15 oz) can kidney beans, rinsed and drained
- 1 cup green lentils, rinsed
- 4 cups vegetable broth
- 2 cups zucchini, chopped

- 1 cup corn kernels (fresh or frozen)
- 2 tbsp chili powder
- 1 tsp cumin
- 1/2 tsp dried oregano
- Salt and freshly ground black pepper, to taste

Optional additions:

- 1 (4 oz) can diced green chilies (for added spiciness)
- 1 cup sliced mushrooms
- 1 bay leaf

ii. For the Sweet Cornbread:

- 1 cup all-purpose flour
- 1 cup yellow cornmeal
- 1/3 cup granulated sugar
- 2 tsp baking powder
- 1/2 tsp salt
- 1 egg, beaten
- 1 1/3 cups milk
- 3 tbsp melted butter

Instructions:

a. Preparing the Chili:

1. Cook the Vegetables: Heat olive oil in a large Dutch oven or pot over medium heat. Add chopped onion, minced garlic, and diced green bell pepper. Sauté until softened, about 5–7 minutes.
2. Incorporate Canned Ingredients: Stir in diced tomatoes with their juices, black beans, kidney beans, and green lentils.
3. Add Broth and Seasonings: Pour in vegetable broth, chili powder, cumin,

dried oregano, salt, and pepper. Include the optional bay leaf (remove before serving). Bring to a boil, then reduce heat, cover, and simmer for 20 minutes.

4. Include Vegetables: Mix in chopped zucchini and corn. Simmer for an additional 10-15 minutes until lentils and vegetables are tender. Optional: Add diced green chilies (if desired) during the final few minutes of cooking.
5. Adjust Seasonings: Taste the chili and adjust seasonings to your preference.

b. Making the Sweet Cornbread:

1. Preheat the Oven: Preheat oven to 400°F (200°C). Grease an 8x8 inch baking pan.
2. Combine Dry Ingredients: In a large bowl, whisk together flour, cornmeal, sugar, baking powder, and salt.
3. Mix Wet Ingredients: In a separate bowl, whisk together beaten egg, milk, and melted butter.
4. Blend and Bake: Pour wet ingredients into dry ingredients and stir just until combined (some lumps are okay). Pour batter into prepared baking pan.
5. Bake: Bake cornbread for 20-25 minutes, or until a toothpick inserted into the center comes out clean.

c. Serving:

- Serve the vegetarian chili in bowls, accompanied by warm slices of sweet cornbread.

Tips:

- Experiment with different bean and vegetable varieties in your chili for variety.

- To thicken the chili, mash some cooked beans against the side of the pot with a fork.
- Store leftover chili in an airtight container in the refrigerator for up to 3 days. Reheat gently on the stovetop. Leftover cornbread can be stored at room temperature for up to 2 days or tightly wrapped and frozen for longer storage.

Greek Salad with Grilled Chicken and Whole-Wheat Pita Bread

Ingredients:

i. For the Salad:

- 2 boneless, skinless chicken breasts or thighs
- 1 tbsp olive oil
- 1 tsp dried oregano
- 1/2 tsp garlic powder
- Salt and freshly ground black pepper, to taste
- 4 cups chopped romaine lettuce or mixed greens
- 1 cucumber, thinly sliced
- 1 tomato, thinly sliced
- 1 red onion, thinly sliced (optional, for added zing)
- 1 cup crumbled feta cheese
- 1/2 cup pitted and halved Kalamata olives
- 1/4 cup chopped fresh parsley
- 2 tbsp red wine vinegar
- 1 tbsp olive oil
- Oregano or lemon-pepper seasoning (optional, for extra flavor)

ii. For Serving:

- 2 whole-wheat pita breads, warmed (optional)

Instructions:

1. Marinating the Chicken (Optional): Combine 1 tablespoon olive oil, oregano, garlic powder, salt, and pepper in a shallow dish. Coat chicken evenly with the marinade. Marinate for at least 15 minutes (or up to 30 minutes for more flavor).
2. Grilling the Chicken: Preheat grill to medium-high heat. Grill chicken for 5-7 minutes per side, until cooked through and golden brown. Alternatively, bake chicken in a preheated oven at 400°F (200°C) for 20-25 minutes, until cooked through.
3. Preparing the Salad: Wash and chop romaine lettuce or mixed greens. Slice cucumber, tomato, and red onion (if using).
4. Assembling the Salad: In a large bowl, combine lettuce/greens, cucumber, tomato, red onion (if using), feta cheese, Kalamata olives, and parsley.
5. Making the Dressing: Whisk together red wine vinegar, olive oil, and a pinch of oregano or lemon-pepper seasoning (optional) for extra flavor.
6. Serving: Slice cooked chicken and arrange over the salad. Drizzle dressing over everything and toss gently to combine.
7. Warming the Pita Bread (Optional): Warm whole-wheat pita breads in a skillet or microwave for a few seconds if desired. Serve salad alongside warmed pita bread for scooping.

Tips:

- Use a grill pan, if an outdoor grill isn't available.
- Experiment with different vegetables in the salad, such as bell peppers or avocado.
- For a creamier dressing, whisk in plain Greek yogurt or tahini to the vinaigrette.

Additional Variations:

- Lemon Herb Infusion: Squeeze fresh lemon juice over the salad for added zest, and sprinkle with chopped fresh herbs like dill or mint.

- Cucumber Refreshment: Substitute pureed cucumber for red wine vinegar in the dressing for a lighter option.
- Spicy Touch: Add a drizzle of sriracha or hot sauce to the dressing for a hint of heat.

Creamy Tomato Pasta with Whole-Wheat Penne

Ingredients:

- 1 tbsp olive oil
- 1 medium onion, finely chopped
- 2 cloves garlic, minced
- 1 (28 oz) can crushed tomatoes, with juices
- 1/2 cup low-sodium chicken broth
- 1/2 cup heavy cream (or opt for low-fat milk or unsweetened almond milk for a lighter version)
- 2 tbsp grated Parmesan cheese
- 1 tsp dried basil
- 1/2 tsp dried oregano
- Pinch of red pepper flakes (optional, for added heat)
- Salt and freshly ground black pepper, to taste
- 1 pound whole-wheat penne pasta
- Fresh chopped parsley, for garnish (optional)

Instructions:

1. Cook the Pasta: Bring a large pot of salted water to a boil. Cook whole-wheat penne according to package instructions for al dente (usually 8–10 minutes). Drain pasta, reserving about 1/2 cup of pasta water.
2. Sauté the Aromatics: In a large skillet or Dutch oven over medium heat, warm olive oil. Add finely chopped onion and cook until softened, about 5–7 minutes. Add minced garlic and cook for another minute until fragrant.

3. Simmer the Tomato Sauce: Stir in crushed tomatoes, chicken broth, heavy cream (or milk alternative), Parmesan cheese, dried basil, oregano, and red pepper flakes (if using). Season with salt and pepper. Bring to a simmer and cook for 10-15 minutes, stirring occasionally to blend flavors.

4. Combine and Adjust Consistency: Add drained whole-wheat penne to the simmering sauce. Gently toss to coat pasta evenly. If sauce is too thick, add a splash of reserved pasta water to achieve desired consistency.

5. Serve and Garnish (Optional): Plate creamy tomato pasta and sprinkle with fresh chopped parsley if desired. Serve hot and enjoy!

Tips:

- Add a pinch of sugar to the sauce to balance tomato acidity.
- For added protein, mix in cooked shredded chicken or crumbled sausage before serving.
- Store leftover pasta in an airtight container in the refrigerator for up to 3 days. Reheat gently on stovetop, adding milk or broth if needed for consistency.

Additional Variations:

- Spinach Addition: Add chopped fresh spinach to sauce during last minute of cooking for a vibrant, nutritious addition.
- Roasted Vegetable Twist: Incorporate roasted vegetables like diced zucchini, bell peppers, or broccoli for extra flavor, color, and fiber.
- Sun-Dried Tomato Infusion: Mix chopped sun-dried tomatoes into the sauce for intensified tomato flavor.

Low-Carb Lunch Options

Chicken Caesar Salad

Ingredients:

i. For the Salad:

- 2 boneless, skinless chicken breasts or thighs
- 1 tbsp olive oil
- 1/2 tsp dried oregano
- 1/4 tsp garlic powder
- Salt and freshly ground black pepper, to taste
- 4 cups chopped romaine lettuce
- 1 cucumber, sliced
- 1/2 red onion, thinly sliced (optional)
- 1 avocado, sliced
- 1/4 cup cherry tomatoes, halved (optional)
- 1/4 cup crumbled parmesan cheese
- Parmesan cheese crisps, for garnish (see recipe below)

ii. For the Caesar Dressing (Low-Carb Option):

- 2 tbsp freshly squeezed lemon juice
- 1 tbsp Dijon mustard
- 1 tbsp tahini (or substitute with 1 tbsp olive oil and 1/2 tsp sesame seeds)
- 1 anchovy fillet (optional, for enhanced umami flavor)
- 1 clove garlic, minced
- 1/4 cup grated parmesan cheese
- 2 tbsp extra virgin olive oil
- Salt and freshly ground black pepper, to taste

Instructions:

1. Marinate the Chicken (Optional): Combine olive oil, oregano, garlic

powder, salt, and pepper in a shallow dish. Coat chicken evenly with the marinade. Marinate for at least 15 minutes (or up to 30 minutes for intensified flavor).

2. Grill or Cook the Chicken: Preheat grill to medium-high heat. Grill chicken for 5-7 minutes per side until cooked through and golden brown. Alternatively, bake chicken in a preheated oven at 400°F (200°C) for 20-25 minutes until done. Once cooked, slice chicken into bite-sized pieces.

3. Prepare the Salad: Wash and chop romaine lettuce. Slice cucumber, red onion (if using), and avocado. Halve cherry tomatoes (optional). Crumble parmesan cheese.

4. Make the Caesar Dressing: In a blender or food processor, blend lemon juice, Dijon mustard, tahini (or olive oil and sesame seeds), anchovy fillet (if using), garlic, parmesan cheese, olive oil, salt, and pepper until smooth and emulsified. Adjust seasonings to taste.

5. Assemble and Serve: In a large bowl, combine chopped romaine lettuce, sliced cucumber, red onion (if using), avocado, cherry tomatoes (if using), and crumbled parmesan cheese. Toss with desired amount of Caesar dressing.

6. Top with Chicken and Crisps: Arrange sliced chicken on top of the salad. Garnish with parmesan cheese crisps for a savory finish.

Parmesan Cheese Crisps (Optional):

- Preheat oven to 375°F (190°C).
- Line a baking sheet with parchment paper.
- Using a cheese slicer or vegetable peeler, create thin parmesan cheese shavings.
- Arrange cheese shavings on prepared baking sheet, leaving space between each crisp.
- Bake for 5-7 minutes until golden brown and edges are melted.
- Let cool completely before using as garnish.

Tips:

- Substitute tahini with a nut butter alternative like cashew or almond butter if unavailable (note: this increases calorie and fat content slightly).
- For a creamier dressing, add a tablespoon of plain Greek yogurt.
- Store leftover grilled chicken in an airtight container in the refrigerator for up to 3 days.

Additional Variations:

- Spicy Twist: Drizzle dressing with sriracha or hot sauce for added heat.
- Herb Infusion: Add chopped fresh herbs like chives or dill for extra flavor dimension.

Grilled Shrimp with Zucchini Noodles and Pesto

Ingredients:

i. For the Shrimp:

- 1 pound large shrimp, peeled and deveined (tails on or off, as preferred)
- 1 tbsp olive oil
- 1/2 tsp dried oregano
- 1/4 tsp garlic powder
- Salt and freshly ground black pepper, to taste

ii. For the Zucchini Noodles:

- 2 medium zucchini
- 1 tbsp olive oil
- Salt and freshly ground black pepper, to taste

iii. For Serving:

- ½ cup prepared pesto (homemade or store-bought)
- Cherry tomatoes, halved (optional)
- Fresh basil leaves, for garnish (optional)

Instructions:

1. Marinate the Shrimp: In a shallow dish, mix olive oil, oregano, garlic powder, salt, and pepper. Add shrimp and toss to coat evenly. Marinate for 15-30 minutes.
2. Prepare the Grill (Optional): If using a grill, preheat to medium-high heat.
3. Spiralize the Zucchini: Create zucchini noodles using a spiralizer or julienne peeler.
4. Sauté the Zucchini Noodles (Optional): In a large skillet, heat olive oil over medium heat. Add zucchini noodles and cook for 2-3 minutes until slightly softened. Season with salt and pepper. Alternatively, serve zucchini noodles raw for extra freshness.
5. Grill or Cook the Shrimp: Grill shrimp on skewers for 2-3 minutes per side until pink and opaque. Alternatively, cook in a skillet over medium heat for the same duration.
6. Assemble and Serve: Divide zucchini noodles among plates. Top with grilled shrimp, a dollop of pesto, and cherry tomatoes if desired. Garnish with fresh basil leaves and serve promptly.

Tips:

- Enhance the shrimp marinade with a teaspoon of smoked paprika for a smoky touch.
- If grilling isn't an option, shrimp can be easily cooked in a skillet.
- Store leftover grilled shrimp in the refrigerator for up to 2 days.

Ham and Swiss Roll-Ups with Mustard on Romaine Lettuce

Ingredients:

- 4-6 slices deli ham (opt for a lower-sodium option if desired)
- 4 slices Swiss cheese
- 2 tbsp Dijon mustard (or your preferred mustard)
- Romaine lettuce leaves, washed and dried

Instructions:

1. Prepare the Roll-Ups: Lay a slice of ham flat on a clean surface. Spread a thin layer of Dijon mustard (or your preferred mustard) evenly over the ham, leaving a small border around the edge.
2. Add Cheese and Roll: Place a slice of Swiss cheese on top of the mustard-covered ham. Roll up the ham and cheese tightly, starting from the short end. Repeat the process with the remaining ham and cheese slices.
3. Assemble and Serve: Arrange the prepared ham and Swiss roll-ups on a platter lined with romaine lettuce leaves. Serve immediately.

Tips:

- For a more vibrant presentation, consider using colorful mustard varieties such as whole-grain Dijon or honey mustard.
- If the ham slices are too large, you can cut them in half before assembling the roll-ups.
- Leftover ham and Swiss roll-ups can be stored in an airtight container in the refrigerator for up to 2 days.

Taco Salad with Ground Beef, Lettuce Wraps, and Pico de Gallo

Ingredients:

i. For the Ground Beef:

- 1 lb lean ground beef (90% lean or higher)
- 1 tbsp olive oil
- 1 medium onion, chopped
- 2 cloves garlic, minced
- 1 tbsp taco seasoning
- 1/2 tsp chili powder (optional, for a touch of heat)
- Salt and freshly ground black pepper, to taste

ii. For the Salad:

- 1 head romaine lettuce, leaves separated and washed
- 1 avocado, sliced (optional)
- 1 tomato, chopped
- 1/2 cup shredded cheddar cheese (optional)
- 1/4 cup crumbled cotija cheese (optional)
- Chopped fresh cilantro, for garnish (optional)

iii. For the Pico de Gallo:

- 1 roma tomato, seeded and diced
- 1/4 cup red onion, diced
- 1 jalapeno pepper, seeded and finely chopped (optional, for a kick of heat)
- 1/4 cup chopped fresh cilantro
- 1 tbsp fresh lime juice
- Salt and freshly ground black pepper, to taste

Instructions:

1. Make the Pico de Gallo: In a small bowl, combine the diced tomato, red onion, jalapeno (if using), chopped cilantro, lime juice, salt, and pepper. Stir well and set aside.

2. Brown the Ground Beef: Heat olive oil in a large skillet over medium heat. Add the ground beef and cook until browned, breaking it up with a spoon. Drain any excess fat.

3. Season the Beef: Stir in the taco seasoning, chili powder (if using), salt, and pepper. Cook for an additional minute to allow flavors to meld.

4. Assemble the Salad: Arrange romaine lettuce leaves on a platter or individual plates. Top with seasoned ground beef, sliced avocado (if using), chopped tomato, shredded cheddar cheese (if using), and crumbled cotija cheese (if using).

5. Serve with Pico de Gallo and Garnish (Optional): Spoon the prepared pico de gallo over the salad or serve it on the side for individual customization. Garnish with chopped fresh cilantro (optional) and serve immediately.

Tips:

- To make the lettuce cups easier to hold, use large romaine lettuce leaves and gently scoop out some of the lettuce from the center to create a bowl-like shape.
- Experiment with different taco seasoning blends or add your own mix of spices for a personalized flavor profile.
- Leftover ground beef can be stored in the refrigerator for up to 3 days. Reheat gently on the stovetop for use in other recipes.

Cobb Salad with Grilled Chicken, Avocado, and Blue Cheese

Ingredients:

i. For the Grilled Chicken:

- 2 boneless, skinless chicken breasts or thighs

- 1 tbsp olive oil
- 1/2 tsp dried oregano
- 1/4 tsp garlic powder
- Salt and freshly ground black pepper, to taste

ii. For the Salad:

- 4 cups romaine lettuce, chopped
- 1 cucumber, sliced
- 1/2 red onion, thinly sliced (optional)
- 1 avocado, sliced
- 1 hard-boiled egg, sliced
- 1/4 cup crumbled blue cheese
- Cherry tomatoes, halved (optional)
- Chopped fresh chives, for garnish (optional)

iii. For the Blue Cheese Dressing (Optional):

- 2 tbsp mayonnaise
- 2 tbsp sour cream
- 1 tbsp buttermilk (or milk thinned with a splash of vinegar or lemon juice)
- 1 tbsp crumbled blue cheese
- 1 tsp lemon juice
- 1/4 tsp Worcestershire sauce
- Salt and freshly ground black pepper, to taste

Instructions:

1. Marinate the Chicken (Optional): In a shallow dish, combine the olive oil, oregano, garlic powder, salt, and pepper. Add the chicken breasts or thighs and coat them evenly with the marinade. Let the chicken marinate for at least 15 minutes (or up to 30 minutes for extra flavor).
2. Grill or Cook the Chicken: Preheat your grill to medium-high heat. Grill

the chicken for 5-7 minutes per side, or until cooked through and golden brown. Alternatively, bake the chicken in a preheated oven at 400°F (200°C) for 20-25 minutes, or until cooked through. Once cooked, slice the chicken into bite-sized pieces.

3. Prepare the Salad: Wash and chop the romaine lettuce. Slice the cucumber, red onion (if using), and avocado. Hard-boil an egg and slice it. Halve the cherry tomatoes (optional). Crumble the blue cheese.

4. Make the Blue Cheese Dressing (Optional): In a small bowl, whisk together the mayonnaise, sour cream, buttermilk, crumbled blue cheese, lemon juice, Worcestershire sauce, salt, and pepper. Taste and adjust seasonings as needed.

5. Assemble and Serve: Arrange the chopped romaine lettuce on a large platter or individual plates. Top with the sliced chicken, cucumber, red onion (if using), avocado, hard-boiled egg slices, and crumbled blue cheese.

6. Drizzle with Dressing (Optional): Drizzle the optional blue cheese dressing over the salad or serve it on the side for individual customization. Garnish with chopped fresh chives (optional) and serve immediately.

Tips:

- If you don't have buttermilk, you can make your own by whisking together 1 tbsp of white vinegar or lemon juice with 1 cup of milk. Let it sit for 5 minutes before using.
- Feel free to add a sprinkle of crumbled bacon bits for a smoky flavor and a touch more protein (be mindful of adding carbs from the bacon).
- Leftover grilled chicken can be stored in an airtight container in the refrigerator for up to 3 days.

Salmon with Cauliflower Rice and Roasted Broccoli

Ingredients:

i. For the Salmon:

- 2 salmon fillets (around 6 oz each), skin on or off (your preference)
- 1 tbsp olive oil
- 1/2 tsp dried dill
- 1/4 tsp garlic powder
- Salt and freshly ground black pepper, to taste

ii. For the Cauliflower Rice:

- 1 head cauliflower, cut into florets
- 1 tbsp olive oil
- 1/2 tsp dried parsley
- Salt and freshly ground black pepper, to taste

iii. For the Roasted Broccoli:

- 1 head broccoli, cut into florets
- 1 tbsp olive oil
- 1/4 tsp garlic powder
- Salt and freshly ground black pepper, to taste

Instructions:

1. Preheat the Oven: Preheat your oven to 400°F (200°C).
2. Prepare the Cauliflower Rice: In a food processor, pulse the cauliflower florets until they resemble rice-sized granules. Alternatively, you can grate the cauliflower using the coarse grater attachment on a box grater.
3. Season the Cauliflower Rice: In a large bowl, toss the cauliflower rice

with olive oil, dried parsley, salt, and pepper.

4. Prepare the Broccoli: In a separate bowl, toss the broccoli florets with olive oil, garlic powder, salt, and pepper.

5. Prepare the Salmon: Pat the salmon fillets dry with paper towels. Season them with olive oil, dried dill, salt, and pepper.

6. Assemble the Sheet Pan: Arrange the cauliflower rice in an even layer on a large baking sheet. Scatter the broccoli florets around the cauliflower rice. Place the seasoned salmon fillets on top of the vegetables.

7. Roast: Bake the sheet pan for 15-20 minutes, or until the salmon is cooked through (flaky with a fork) and the vegetables are tender-crisp.

8. Serve: Divide the roasted vegetables and salmon among plates and serve immediately.

Tips:

- For a bit of a crispy skin on the salmon, place the fillets skin-side down on the baking sheet during the first half of roasting, then flip them over for the last few minutes.
- If you don't have a food processor, you can use a box grater with the coarse grater attachment to create the cauliflower rice.

Turkey Lettuce Wraps with Asian Slaw

Ingredients:

i. For the Turkey Filling:

- 1 pound ground turkey (90% lean or higher)
- 1 tbsp olive oil
- 1 onion, chopped
- 2 cloves garlic, minced
- 1 tbsp soy sauce, low-sodium preferred
- 1 tbsp rice vinegar

- 1 tbsp grated ginger
- 1 tsp Sriracha (or to taste, for a kick of heat)
- 1/2 tsp sesame oil
- Salt and freshly ground black pepper, to taste

ii. For the Asian Slaw:

- 2 cups shredded cabbage (green or Napa)
- 1 carrot, julienned (or shredded)
- 1/2 cup chopped fresh cilantro
- 2 tbsp rice vinegar
- 1 tbsp soy sauce, low-sodium preferred
- 1 tbsp sesame oil
- 1 tsp honey (or maple syrup for a vegan option)
- Salt and freshly ground black pepper, to taste

iii. For Serving:

- 1 head romaine lettuce leaves, washed and separated
- Chopped peanuts (optional, for garnish)
- Sesame seeds (optional, for garnish)

Instructions:

1. Make the Asian Slaw: In a large bowl, combine the shredded cabbage, julienned carrots, and chopped cilantro.
2. Whisk the Dressing: In a small bowl, whisk together the rice vinegar, soy sauce, sesame oil, honey (or maple syrup), salt, and pepper. Pour the dressing over the slaw mixture and toss to coat evenly. Set aside.
3. Brown the Ground Turkey: In a large skillet over medium heat, heat the olive oil. Add the ground turkey and cook, breaking it up with a spoon, until browned. Drain any excess fat.
4. Season the Turkey: Stir in the chopped onion, minced garlic, soy sauce,

rice vinegar, grated ginger, Sriracha (if using), and sesame oil. Cook for an additional minute, allowing the flavors to meld. Season with salt and pepper to taste.

5. Assemble and Serve: Arrange the romaine lettuce leaves on a platter or individual plates. Fill each lettuce leaf with a portion of the seasoned ground turkey. Top with the Asian slaw.

6. Garnish (Optional): Sprinkle with chopped peanuts and sesame seeds (optional) and serve immediately.

Tips:

- To make lettuce wraps easier to hold and fill, use large romaine lettuce leaves and gently scoop out some of the lettuce from the center to create a more bowl-like shape.
- Feel free to adjust the amount of Sriracha to your preferred level of spiciness.
- Leftover ground turkey filling can be stored in an airtight container in the refrigerator for up to 3 days. Repurpose it in other recipes like stuffed peppers or stir-fries.

Soup and Salad (Split Pea Soup with Side Salad)

Ingredients:

i. For the Split Pea Soup:

- 1 tbsp olive oil
- 1 onion, chopped
- 2 carrots, chopped
- 2 celery stalks, chopped
- 2 cloves garlic, minced
- 1 tsp dried thyme
- 1/2 tsp dried rosemary

- 1/4 tsp black pepper
- 1 cup dried green split peas, rinsed
- 4 cups low-sodium chicken broth
- 2 cups water
- 1 bay leaf

ii. For the Side Salad:

- 2 cups mixed greens, washed and dried
- 1/2 cucumber, sliced
- 1/4 cup cherry tomatoes, halved
- 2 tbsp crumbled feta cheese (optional)
- 2 tbsp olive oil and vinegar dressing (or your favorite low-carb dressing)

Instructions:

1. Sauté the Aromatics: Heat olive oil in a large pot over medium heat. Add onion, carrots, and celery. Sauté for 5-7 minutes until softened. Stir in garlic, thyme, rosemary, and black pepper. Cook for 1 minute.
2. Add Split Peas and Broth: Add rinsed split peas, chicken broth, water, and bay leaf to the pot. Bring to a boil, then reduce heat and simmer for 45-60 minutes until split peas are tender and soup has thickened.
3. Remove Bay Leaf and Mash (Optional): Remove bay leaf. For a smoother texture, partially mash some of the soup using an immersion blender or food processor.
4. Prepare the Side Salad: Arrange mixed greens on a plate. Top with sliced cucumber, cherry tomatoes, and crumbled feta cheese (if using). Drizzle with your favorite low-carb salad dressing.
5. Serve: Ladle split pea soup into bowls and serve alongside the prepared side salad. Enjoy hot!

Tips:

- Add other vegetables to the soup, such as chopped potatoes or green beans, for extra flavor and fiber (be mindful of extra carbs with potatoes).
- Stir in chopped fresh parsley or dill to the finished soup for a richer flavor.
- Store leftover split pea soup in an airtight container in the refrigerator for up to 3 days. Reheat gently on the stovetop.

Beef Stir-Fry with Broccoli and Snow Peas over Cauliflower Rice

Ingredients:

i. For the Beef Stir-Fry:

- 1 lb flank steak or skirt steak, thinly sliced against the grain
- 1 tbsp cornstarch (or arrowroot powder for a gluten-free option)
- 2 tbsp low-sodium soy sauce
- 1 tbsp rice vinegar
- 1 tbsp sesame oil
- 1/2 tsp grated ginger
- 1 clove garlic, minced
- 1 tbsp vegetable oil
- 1 head broccoli, cut into florets
- 1 cup snow peas
- 1/4 cup chopped green onions

ii. For the Cauliflower Rice:

- 1 head cauliflower, cut into florets
- 1 tbsp olive oil
- Salt and freshly ground black pepper, to taste

Instructions:

1. Marinate the Beef: In a shallow bowl, combine sliced beef with cornstarch,

soy sauce, rice vinegar, sesame oil, grated ginger, and minced garlic. Toss to coat evenly. Marinate for at least 15 minutes (or up to 30 minutes for extra flavor).

2. Prepare the Cauliflower Rice: In a food processor, pulse cauliflower florets until rice-sized granules form. Alternatively, grate cauliflower using a box grater.

3. Cook the Cauliflower Rice: Heat olive oil in a large skillet or wok over medium heat. Add cauliflower rice and cook for 3-5 minutes until slightly softened. Season with salt and pepper. Set aside.

4. Stir-Fry the Beef: Heat vegetable oil in a separate wok or large skillet over high heat. Add marinated beef (discard marinade). Stir-fry for 2-3 minutes until browned and cooked through. Remove from pan and set aside.

5. Stir-Fry the Vegetables: Add broccoli florets and snow peas to the same pan. Stir-fry for 3-4 minutes until crisp-tender.

6. Assemble and Serve: Return cooked beef to the pan with vegetables. Toss to combine and heat through for 1 minute.

7. Plate and Garnish: Divide cauliflower rice among plates. Top with stir-fried beef and vegetables. Garnish with chopped green onions and serve immediately.

Tips:

- Slice beef thinly against the grain for tenderness.
- Substitute arrowroot powder for cornstarch if needed.
- Store leftover stir-fry in an airtight container in the refrigerator for up to 3 days.

Tuna Salad with Mixed Greens and Avocado

Ingredients:

i. For the Tuna Salad:

- 2 (5 oz) cans tuna packed in water, drained and flaked
- 1/4 cup mayonnaise (or plain Greek yogurt for a lighter option)
- 1 celery stalk, finely chopped
- 1/4 red onion, finely chopped (optional)
- 1 tablespoon lemon juice
- 1 tablespoon chopped fresh parsley
- 1/4 teaspoon dried dill
- Salt and freshly ground black pepper, to taste

ii. For the Salad:

- 4 cups mixed greens, washed and dried
- 1 ripe avocado, sliced
- Cherry tomatoes, halved (optional)
- 2 tablespoons olive oil and vinegar dressing (or your favorite low-carb dressing)

Instructions:

1. Prepare the Tuna Salad: In a medium bowl, mix together the flaked tuna, mayonnaise (or Greek yogurt), chopped celery, red onion (if using), lemon juice, chopped parsley, dried dill, salt, and pepper. Combine well.
2. Assemble the Salad: Arrange the mixed greens on a large platter or individual plates. Top with sliced avocado and cherry tomatoes, if desired.
3. Add Tuna Salad: Spoon the prepared tuna salad over the bed of greens.
4. Serve: Drizzle the salad with your preferred low-carb dressing and serve immediately.

Tips:

- For extra creaminess, mash some avocado into the tuna salad mixture.
- If fresh herbs are unavailable, substitute with 1/2 teaspoon dried parsley and 1/4 teaspoon dried dill.

- Leftover tuna salad can be refrigerated in an airtight container for up to 2 days. Serve leftovers on romaine lettuce wraps or cucumber slices for a different low-carb option.

5

Chapter 5

Dinner Recipes

High-Carb Dinner Options

Baked Chicken with Sweet Potato Mash and Green Beans

Ingredients:

i. For the Baked Chicken:

- 4 boneless, skinless chicken breasts or thighs (approximately 6 oz each)
- 2 tablespoons olive oil
- 1 tablespoon dried thyme
- 1/2 teaspoon garlic powder
- 1/2 teaspoon paprika
- Salt and freshly ground black pepper, to taste

ii. For the Sweet Potato Mash:

- 2 large sweet potatoes, peeled and cubed
- 1/2 cup low-sodium chicken broth
- 1 tablespoon butter
- 1/4 cup milk (or unsweetened almond milk)
- Salt and freshly ground black pepper, to taste
- Pinch of freshly grated nutmeg (optional)

iii. For the Green Beans:

- 1 pound fresh green beans, trimmed
- 1 tablespoon olive oil
- 1/4 cup water
- Salt and freshly ground black pepper, to taste

Instructions:

1. Preheat the Oven: Preheat the oven to 400°F (200°C).
2. Marinate the Chicken (Optional): In a shallow dish, mix the olive oil, dried thyme, garlic powder, paprika, salt, and pepper. Coat the chicken breasts or thighs evenly with the marinade. Marinate for at least 15 minutes, or up to 30 minutes for more flavor.
3. Boil the Sweet Potatoes: Place the cubed sweet potatoes in a medium saucepan, cover with water, and bring to a boil. Reduce the heat and simmer for 10-15 minutes, until the sweet potatoes are tender. Drain the water.
4. Mash the Sweet Potatoes: While the sweet potatoes are still hot, mash them using a potato masher or immersion blender. Add the chicken broth, butter, milk (or almond milk), salt, pepper, and nutmeg (if using). Mix until smooth and creamy. Set aside.
5. Prepare the Green Beans: In a large skillet, heat olive oil over medium heat. Add the green beans and water. Season with salt and pepper. Cover and steam for 5-7 minutes, until the green beans are tender-crisp.
6. Bake the Chicken: Place the marinated chicken breasts or thighs on a

baking sheet. Bake for 20-25 minutes, until the chicken is cooked through and juices run clear.

7. Assemble and Serve: Divide the sweet potato mash and green beans among plates. Place a baked chicken breast or thigh on each plate. Serve hot.

Tips:

- For crispier chicken skin, broil the chicken for the last 2-3 minutes of baking, but monitor closely to prevent burning.
- Substitute dried thyme with dried oregano or Italian seasoning if needed.
- Leftovers can be stored in an airtight container in the refrigerator for up to 3 days. Reheat gently before serving.

Shrimp Scampi with Whole-Wheat Pasta

Ingredients:

i. For the Shrimp Scampi:

- 1 pound large shrimp, peeled and deveined (tails on or off)
- 2 tablespoons olive oil
- 4 cloves garlic, minced
- 1/2 teaspoon red pepper flakes (optional)
- 1/2 cup dry white wine (chardonnay or sauvignon blanc)
- 1/2 cup low-sodium chicken broth
- 1/2 cup heavy cream
- 2 tablespoons fresh lemon juice
- 1 tablespoon chopped fresh parsley
- Salt and freshly ground black pepper, to taste

ii. For the Whole-Wheat Pasta:

- 8 ounces whole-wheat spaghetti or preferred whole-wheat pasta shape
- Salt

Instructions:

1. Cook the Pasta: Bring a large pot of salted water to a boil. Add the whole-wheat pasta and cook according to package instructions for al dente texture (usually 8-10 minutes). Reserve about 1/4 cup of pasta cooking water before draining.
2. Prepare the Shrimp Scampi: Pat the shrimp dry with paper towels. Heat olive oil in a large skillet over medium heat.
3. Sauté Garlic and Red Pepper Flakes: Add minced garlic and red pepper flakes (if using) to the hot oil. Sauté for 30 seconds until fragrant, being cautious not to burn the garlic.
4. Sear the Shrimp: Add shrimp to the skillet and cook for 1-2 minutes per side until pink and opaque. Remove cooked shrimp from the skillet and set aside.
5. Deglaze the Pan: Pour white wine into the skillet, scraping up any browned bits. Simmer for a minute or two to cook off the alcohol.
6. Add Broth, Cream, and Lemon Juice: Stir in chicken broth, heavy cream, and lemon juice. Simmer for 2-3 minutes until the sauce slightly thickens.
7. Return Shrimp and Pasta: Add cooked shrimp and reserved pasta water to the skillet with the sauce. Toss gently to combine and heat through for 1 minute.
8. Serve: Divide pasta and shrimp scampi mixture among plates. Garnish with chopped parsley and serve immediately.

Tips:

- Enhance the sauce's richness by substituting half the heavy cream with unsalted butter.
- If white wine is unavailable, use chicken broth as an alternative.
- Avoid overcooking the shrimp to prevent toughness.

Vegetarian Lasagna with Zucchini Noodles

Ingredients:

i. For the Zucchini Noodles:

- 2 medium zucchini
- 1 tablespoon olive oil
- Salt and freshly ground black pepper, to taste

ii. For the Ricotta Cheese Mixture:

- 15-ounce container ricotta cheese
- 1/2 cup grated Parmesan cheese
- 1 large egg
- 1/4 cup chopped fresh basil
- Salt and freshly ground black pepper, to taste

iii. For the Tomato Sauce:

- 2 tablespoons olive oil
- 1 onion, chopped
- 2 cloves garlic, minced
- 1 (28-ounce) can crushed tomatoes
- 1 tablespoon tomato paste
- 1/2 teaspoon dried oregano
- 1/4 teaspoon red pepper flakes (optional)
- Salt and freshly ground black pepper, to taste
- 1/4 cup shredded mozzarella cheese (optional, for topping)

Instructions:

1. Preheat the Oven: Preheat your oven to 375°F (190°C). Grease a 9x13 inch

baking dish lightly.

2. Prepare the Zucchini Noodles: Create zucchini noodles using a spiralizer or mandoline. Alternatively, thinly slice the zucchini lengthwise.

3. Season and Sauté the Zucchini Noodles: Heat olive oil in a large skillet over medium heat. Add zucchini noodles and cook for 2-3 minutes until slightly softened. Season with salt and pepper, then drain excess moisture using a colander.

4. Make the Ricotta Cheese Mixture: Combine ricotta cheese, Parmesan cheese, egg, chopped basil, salt, and pepper in a bowl. Stir until creamy and well combined.

5. Prepare the Tomato Sauce: Heat olive oil in a large skillet over medium heat. Sauté chopped onion for 5 minutes until softened. Add minced garlic and cook for another minute.

6. Simmer the Sauce: Stir in crushed tomatoes, tomato paste, oregano, and red pepper flakes (if using). Season with salt and pepper. Simmer for 15-20 minutes until the sauce thickens.

7. Assemble the Lasagna: Spread a thin layer of tomato sauce on the bottom of the baking dish. Layer zucchini noodles, followed by half of the ricotta cheese mixture. Repeat with another layer of sauce, noodles, and remaining ricotta mixture.

8. Optional Topping: Sprinkle shredded mozzarella cheese over the top layer if desired.

9. Bake: Bake the lasagna for 25-30 minutes until bubbly and the top is golden brown.

10. Serve: Allow the lasagna to cool slightly before slicing and serving. Enjoy the comforting flavors!

Tips:

- Prevent excess moisture in zucchini noodles by salting and draining them before cooking.
- Enhance the ricotta mixture by adding crumbled whole-wheat bread for richness.

Lentil Shepherd's Pie with Mashed Potatoes

Ingredients:

i. For the Lentil Filling:

- 1 tablespoon olive oil
- 1 onion, chopped
- 2 carrots, chopped
- 2 celery stalks, chopped
- 2 cloves garlic, minced
- 1 cup brown lentils, rinsed
- 4 cups vegetable broth
- 1 (14.5 oz) can diced tomatoes, undrained
- 1 tablespoon tomato paste
- 1 tablespoon Worcestershire sauce (vegetarian or vegan option if needed)
- 1 teaspoon dried thyme
- 1/2 teaspoon dried rosemary
- Salt and freshly ground black pepper, to taste
- 1 cup frozen peas

ii. For the Mashed Potatoes:

- 4–5 russet potatoes, peeled and cut into cubes
- 1/2 cup milk (or unsweetened almond milk)
- 2 tablespoons butter
- Salt and freshly ground black pepper, to taste
- 1/4 cup chopped fresh parsley (optional, for garnish)

Instructions:

1. Preheat the Oven: Preheat your oven to 400°F (200°C). Grease a 9x13 inch baking dish lightly.

2. Sauté the Vegetables: Heat olive oil in a large pot over medium heat. Add chopped onion, carrots, and celery. Sauté for 5-7 minutes until softened. Stir in minced garlic and cook for another minute.

3. Cook Lentils with Broth and Tomatoes: Add rinsed lentils, vegetable broth, diced tomatoes, tomato paste, Worcestershire sauce, dried thyme, and dried rosemary to the pot. Season with salt and pepper. Bring to a boil, then simmer for 20-25 minutes until lentils are tender.

4. Add Peas: Stir frozen peas into the lentil mixture and cook for an additional minute until heated through.

5. Prepare Mashed Potatoes: Boil cubed potatoes in salted water until tender. Drain and mash with milk, butter, salt, and pepper until creamy.

6. Assemble and Bake: Transfer lentil filling to the baking dish. Top with mashed potatoes, spreading evenly.

7. Bake: Bake shepherd's pie for 20-25 minutes until edges are bubbly and top is golden brown.

8. Serve: Let it cool slightly, garnish with chopped parsley if desired, and serve warm!

Tips:

- Mash some cooked lentils for a thicker filling.
- Substitute vegetable broth with low-sodium chicken broth if needed.
- Store leftovers in the refrigerator for up to 3 days and reheat before serving.

Black Bean and Corn Quesadillas with Avocado Crema

Ingredients:

i. For the Black Bean and Corn Filling:

- 1 tablespoon olive oil
- 1 onion, chopped
- 1 clove garlic, minced

- 1 (15 oz) can black beans, rinsed and drained
- 1 cup frozen corn, thawed
- 1/2 cup chopped fresh cilantro
- 1/4 cup shredded cheddar cheese (or your favorite cheese)
- 1/4 teaspoon chili powder
- 1/4 teaspoon cumin
- Salt and freshly ground black pepper, to taste

ii. For the Quesadillas:

- 4 large flour tortillas
- Cooking spray or butter

iii. For the Avocado Crema:

- 1 ripe avocado, pitted and peeled
- 1/4 cup sour cream (or plain Greek yogurt for a lighter option)
- 1 tablespoon lime juice
- 1/4 cup chopped fresh cilantro
- Salt and freshly ground black pepper, to taste

Instructions:

1. Prepare the Black Bean and Corn Filling: Heat olive oil in a large skillet over medium heat. Add chopped onion and cook for 5 minutes until softened. Stir in minced garlic and cook for 1 minute.
2. Add Black Beans, Corn, and Spices: Add black beans, thawed corn, chopped cilantro, shredded cheese, chili powder, cumin, salt, and pepper to the skillet. Stir well and cook for 2-3 minutes.
3. Assemble the Quesadillas: Lay a tortilla flat and coat one half with cooking spray or butter. Spoon a generous portion of the black bean and corn filling onto the coated half. Fold the tortilla in half, pressing gently.
4. Cook Quesadillas: Heat a skillet over medium heat. Place the folded

quesadilla onto the skillet and cook for 2-3 minutes on each side until golden brown and crispy. Repeat with remaining tortillas and filling.

5. Make the Avocado Crema: In a blender or food processor, combine avocado, sour cream (or Greek yogurt), lime juice, chopped cilantro, salt, and pepper. Blend until smooth and creamy.

6. Serve: Cut quesadillas into wedges and serve warm with avocado crema for dipping.

Tips:

- For extra cheese, sprinkle some shredded cheese on top of the filling before folding the tortilla.
- Dried cilantro can be used as a substitute for fresh cilantro.
- Store leftover quesadillas in an airtight container in the refrigerator and reheat before serving.

Teriyaki Salmon with Brown Rice and Edamame

Ingredients:

i. For the Teriyaki Salmon:

- 4 (5-6 oz) salmon fillets
- 1/4 cup low-sodium soy sauce
- 2 tablespoons mirin (or substitute with brown sugar)
- 1 tablespoon honey
- 1 tablespoon rice vinegar
- 1 tablespoon sake (optional)
- 1 clove garlic, minced
- 1 teaspoon grated ginger
- 1 tablespoon cornstarch
- 1 tablespoon water

ii. For the Brown Rice:

- 1 cup brown rice, rinsed
- 1 ½ cups water
- Salt

iii. For the Edamame:

- 1 cup frozen shelled edamame, thawed
- 1 tablespoon olive oil
- 1/4 teaspoon sea salt

Instructions:

1. Marinate the Salmon: Combine soy sauce, mirin (or brown sugar), honey, rice vinegar, sake (if using), minced garlic, and grated ginger in a shallow dish. Add salmon fillets, ensuring they're evenly coated. Marinate for 15-30 minutes.
2. Cook the Brown Rice: In a saucepan, combine rinsed brown rice, water, and a pinch of salt. Bring to a boil, then simmer for 45-50 minutes until rice is fluffy and cooked.
3. Prepare the Edamame: Heat olive oil in a skillet over medium heat. Add thawed edamame and sprinkle with sea salt. Sauté for 3-4 minutes until heated through and slightly blistered.
4. Cook the Salmon: Heat a skillet or grill pan over medium heat. Remove salmon from marinade (reserve marinade) and sear for 3-4 minutes per side until cooked through.
5. Make the Teriyaki Glaze: In a saucepan, heat reserved marinade. Simmer for 2-3 minutes, then add cornstarch and water mixture (cornstarch slurry). Cook until thickened.
6. Assemble and Serve: Divide cooked brown rice among plates. Top with teriyaki salmon and spoon glaze over. Serve with sautéed edamame on the side. Enjoy!

Tips:

- Ensure tender salmon by not overcooking it; it's done when it flakes easily with a fork.
- Substitute brown sugar for mirin if needed.
- Store leftovers in the refrigerator for up to 3 days and reheat before serving.

Turkey Chili with Cornbread Stuffing

Ingredients:

i. For the Turkey Chili:

- 1 tablespoon olive oil
- 1 onion, chopped
- 2 carrots, chopped
- 2 celery stalks, chopped
- 2 cloves garlic, minced
- 1 pound ground turkey
- 1 (15 oz) can diced tomatoes, undrained
- 4 cups low-sodium chicken broth
- 1 (15 oz) can kidney beans, drained and rinsed
- 1 (15 oz) can black beans, drained and rinsed
- 1 cup frozen corn
- 1 tablespoon chili powder
- 1 teaspoon ground cumin
- 1/2 teaspoon dried oregano
- 1/4 teaspoon smoked paprika
- Salt and freshly ground black pepper, to taste

ii. For the Cornbread Stuffing:

- 1 box (8.5 oz) cornbread stuffing mix

- 1/4 cup chopped onion (optional)
- 1/4 cup chopped celery (optional)
- 1/4 cup melted butter
- 1/2 cup chicken broth

Instructions:

1. Brown the Ground Turkey: Heat olive oil in a large pot over medium heat. Add ground turkey and cook until browned. Drain excess grease.
2. Sauté the Vegetables: Add onion, carrots, and celery to the pot with turkey. Sauté until softened. Stir in minced garlic and cook for another minute.
3. Add Beans, Tomatoes, and Broth: Mix in diced tomatoes, kidney beans, black beans, frozen corn, chicken broth, chili powder, cumin, oregano, smoked paprika, salt, and pepper. Stir well.
4. Simmer the Chili: Bring the chili to a boil, then reduce heat and simmer for 30-40 minutes until flavors meld and chili thickens slightly.
5. Prepare the Cornbread Stuffing (Optional): Preheat oven to 375°F (190°C). In a bowl, combine cornbread stuffing mix, chopped onion (if using), chopped celery (if using), melted butter, and chicken broth. Stir until moist stuffing forms.
6. Assemble and Bake (Optional): If using cornbread stuffing, spoon chili into a baking dish. Spread cornbread stuffing evenly over chili. Bake for 20-25 minutes until stuffing is golden brown and crispy.
7. Serve: Ladle turkey chili into bowls. If using cornbread stuffing, serve immediately. If not, serve chili hot with optional toppings.

Tips:

- For thicker chili, mash some cooked beans before adding back to pot.
- Adjust spice level to taste; add red pepper flakes for heat.
- Store leftovers in fridge for up to 3 days; reheat on stovetop.

One-Pot Chicken and Veggie Paella

Ingredients:

- 1 tablespoon olive oil
- 1 medium onion, chopped
- 1 bell pepper (red, yellow, or orange), chopped
- 2 cloves garlic, minced
- 1 pound boneless, skinless chicken thighs, cut into bite-sized pieces
- 1 (14.5 oz) can diced tomatoes, undrained
- 1 cup chicken broth
- 1 1/2 cups long-grain white rice
- 1 teaspoon paprika
- 1/2 teaspoon dried thyme
- Pinch of saffron threads (optional)
- 1 cup frozen peas
- 1/2 cup chopped fresh parsley
- Salt and freshly ground black pepper, to taste

Instructions:

1. Sauté the Vegetables: Heat olive oil in a large Dutch oven or oven-safe pot over medium heat. Add chopped onion and bell pepper. Sauté until softened, about 5-7 minutes. Stir in minced garlic and cook for another minute.
2. Sear the Chicken: Add chicken pieces to the pot and cook until browned on all sides, about 5-7 minutes.
3. Deglaze the Pan: Pour in diced tomatoes (undrained) and scrape up any browned bits from the bottom of the pot with a wooden spoon.
4. Add Broth, Rice, and Spices: Stir in chicken broth, white rice, paprika, dried thyme, and saffron threads (if using). Season with salt and pepper. Bring to a boil, then reduce heat to low, cover, and simmer for 15 minutes.
5. Stir in Peas: After 15 minutes, stir in frozen peas. Continue to simmer,

covered, for an additional 5 minutes until rice is cooked through and peas are heated.

6. Fluff and Garnish: Remove from heat and let it stand for 5 minutes. Fluff rice with a fork before serving. Sprinkle with chopped fresh parsley for garnish.

7. Serve: Enjoy the one-pot chicken and veggie paella hot!

Whole-Wheat Pasta Primavera with Seasonal Vegetables

Ingredients:

i. For the Pasta:

- 8 ounces whole-wheat penne pasta (or preferred whole-wheat pasta shape)
- Salt

ii. For the Vegetables:

- 1 tablespoon olive oil
- 1 small onion, chopped
- 2 cloves garlic, minced
- 1 cup asparagus spears, trimmed and cut into bite-sized pieces
- 1 cup sugar snap peas, trimmed and halved (or snow peas)
- 1 cup cherry tomatoes, halved
- 1 red bell pepper, sliced
- 1 zucchini, sliced
- 1/2 cup shelled fresh peas (or frozen peas, thawed)
- 1/4 cup chopped fresh parsley
- Salt and freshly ground black pepper, to taste

iii. For the Sauce (Optional):

- 1/4 cup low-sodium vegetable broth
- 1 tablespoon lemon juice
- 1 tablespoon grated Parmesan cheese (or vegan cheese alternative)
- 1/4 teaspoon dried oregano
- Pinch of red pepper flakes (optional)

Instructions:

1. Cook the Pasta: Boil a large pot of salted water. Add whole-wheat pasta and cook until al dente. Reserve 1/4 cup of pasta cooking water before draining.
2. Prepare the Vegetables: In a large skillet or Dutch oven, heat olive oil over medium heat. Sauté chopped onion and minced garlic until softened, about 3-4 minutes.
3. Sauté the Seasonal Vegetables: Add asparagus, sugar snap peas (or snow peas), cherry tomatoes, red bell pepper, and zucchini. Sauté until tender-crisp and lightly browned, about 5-7 minutes.
4. Incorporate Peas and Herbs: Stir in fresh peas and chopped parsley. Cook for another minute until peas are heated through.
5. Optional Sauce: Whisk together vegetable broth, lemon juice, grated Parmesan cheese (or vegan alternative), dried oregano, and red pepper flakes (if using).
6. Assemble and Serve: Toss cooked pasta with sautéed vegetables in the skillet. Add optional sauce and toss to combine. Season with salt and black pepper to taste.
7. Serve: Divide pasta primavera among plates and enjoy the burst of flavors!

Tips:

- Enhance flavor with a tablespoon of butter or vegan butter while sautéing vegetables.
- Adjust heat if vegetables release excess moisture; increase slightly to

evaporate.

- Aim for slightly crisp vegetables; avoid overcooking.

Seasonal Swaps:

- **Spring:** Asparagus, sugar snap peas, peas, cherry tomatoes
- **Summer:** Zucchini, yellow squash, corn kernels, bell peppers, fresh basil
- **Fall:** Butternut squash, Brussels sprouts, mushrooms, leafy greens
- **Winter:** Broccoli, cauliflower, sweet potato, carrots

Additional Variations:

- **Protein Boost:** Add grilled chicken, shrimp, or crumbled tofu.
- **Creamy Delight:** Stir in 1/4 cup heavy cream or vegan cream alternative for richness.

Creamy Chicken and Mushroom Risotto

Ingredients:

For the Risotto:

- 1 tablespoon olive oil
- 1 onion, chopped
- 2 cloves garlic, minced
- 1 pound boneless, skinless chicken thighs, cut into bite-sized pieces
- 8 ounces sliced mushrooms (cremini, portobello, or a mix)
- 1 cup Arborio rice
- 1/2 cup dry white wine (chardonnay or sauvignon blanc)
- 4 cups low-sodium chicken broth (warmed)
- 1/2 cup grated Parmesan cheese
- 2 tablespoons unsalted butter
- 1/4 cup chopped fresh parsley

- Salt and freshly ground black pepper, to taste

Instructions:

1. Sauté the Onion and Garlic: Heat olive oil in a large saucepan over medium heat. Sauté chopped onion for 5 minutes until softened. Add minced garlic and cook for another minute.
2. Sear the Chicken: Add chicken pieces to the pot and cook for 5–7 minutes until browned on all sides.
3. Add Mushrooms: Stir in sliced mushrooms and cook for 3–4 minutes until softened and juicy.
4. Toast the Rice: Add Arborio rice to the pan, stirring to coat with oil and vegetables. Cook for 1-2 minutes to toast the rice grains.
5. Deglaze with Wine: Pour in white wine, stirring constantly until almost absorbed.
6. Gradual Broth Addition: Begin adding warmed chicken broth, about ½ cup at a time, stirring frequently until absorbed. Continue for 20-25 minutes until rice is creamy yet al dente.
7. Final Touches: Stir in grated Parmesan cheese, butter, and chopped parsley. Season with salt and pepper to taste.
8. Serve: Enjoy the creamy chicken and mushroom risotto immediately while hot.

Tips:

- Use warm broth to maintain cooking consistency.
- For a richer flavor, replace half the broth with heavy cream.
- Avoid overcooking rice; aim for creamy texture with a slight bite.
- Store leftovers in an airtight container in the refrigerator for up to 2 days.

Additional Variations:

- Spinach Delight: Add 1 cup chopped fresh spinach during the last minute of cooking.

- Herb Delight: Sprinkle chopped fresh thyme or chives over the finished dish for added flavor.

Low-Carb Dinner Options

Salmon with Roasted Brussels Sprouts and Lemon Butter

Ingredients:

i. For the Salmon:

  - 2 (5-6 oz) salmon fillets
  - 1 tablespoon olive oil
  - Salt and freshly ground black pepper, to taste

ii. For the Roasted Brussels Sprouts:

  - 1 pound Brussels sprouts, trimmed and halved
  - 1 tablespoon olive oil
  - 1/2 teaspoon dried thyme
  - Salt and freshly ground black pepper, to taste

iii. For the Lemon Butter (Optional):

  - 4 tablespoons unsalted butter, softened
  - 1 tablespoon lemon juice
  - 1 teaspoon chopped fresh parsley (optional)

Instructions:

1. Preheat the Oven: Preheat your oven to 400°F (200°C). Lightly grease a baking sheet.

2. Prepare the Brussels Sprouts: In a medium bowl, toss halved Brussels sprouts with olive oil, dried thyme, salt, and pepper. Spread them on the prepared baking sheet in a single layer.

3. Roast the Brussels Sprouts: Roast Brussels sprouts for 20-25 minutes until tender-crisp and slightly browned, tossing them halfway through cooking.

4. Season the Salmon: Pat dry salmon fillets with paper towels. Season them generously with salt and pepper.

5. Sear the Salmon (Optional): Heat a large skillet over medium heat. Add a drizzle of olive oil (if needed). Place salmon fillets skin-side down in the hot skillet. Sear for 2-3 minutes until the skin becomes crispy.

6. Bake the Salmon: Transfer seared salmon fillets to a baking dish or baking sheet. Place the baking dish with the salmon in the preheated oven for 8-10 minutes until salmon is cooked through and flakes easily with a fork.

7. Make the Lemon Butter (Optional): In a small bowl, mash together softened butter, lemon juice, and chopped fresh parsley until well combined.

8. Assemble and Serve: Plate roasted Brussels sprouts. Top with cooked salmon fillets. Drizzle with prepared lemon butter (if using) and enjoy!

Tips:

- Ensure perfectly cooked salmon by avoiding overcooking. Salmon is ready when the flesh becomes opaque and flakes easily with a fork.
- Substitute fresh parsley with a pinch of dried parsley flakes if unavailable.
- Store leftovers in an airtight container in the refrigerator for up to 3 days. Reheat gently in the oven or microwave.

Steak Fajitas with Cauliflower Tortillas and Guacamole

Ingredients:

i. For the Steak Fajitas:

- 1 pound flank steak, thinly sliced against the grain
- 1 tablespoon olive oil
- 1 onion, thinly sliced
- 1 bell pepper (red, yellow, or orange), thinly sliced
- 1 teaspoon chili powder
- 1/2 teaspoon ground cumin
- 1/4 teaspoon smoked paprika
- Salt and freshly ground black pepper, to taste

ii. For the Cauliflower Tortillas (makes about 4-6 tortillas):

- 1 head of cauliflower, riced (or 2 cups pre-riced cauliflower)
- 1 large egg
- 1/4 cup shredded mozzarella cheese
- 1/4 cup almond flour (or coconut flour)
- Pinch of salt

iii. For the Guacamole:

- 1 ripe avocado, mashed
- 1/4 cup chopped red onion
- 1 tablespoon chopped fresh cilantro
- Juice of 1/2 lime
- Salt and freshly ground black pepper, to taste

Instructions:

1. Marinate the Steak (Optional): In a large bowl, combine sliced steak with 1 tablespoon olive oil, chili powder, cumin, smoked paprika, salt, and pepper. Toss to coat and marinate for at least 30 minutes or up to overnight for extra flavor (optional).
2. Prepare the Cauliflower Tortillas: Rice the cauliflower florets using a food processor or box grater. In a large bowl, combine riced cauliflower with egg, shredded mozzarella cheese, almond flour (or coconut flour), and a pinch of salt. Mix well to form a cohesive dough.
3. Cook the Cauliflower Tortillas: Heat a lightly oiled skillet over medium heat. Form cauliflower dough into small, thin patties (about 3-4 inches in diameter). Cook for 2-3 minutes per side until golden brown and crispy. Set aside and keep warm.
4. Cook the Steak Fajitas: Heat a large skillet or grill pan over medium-high heat. Add a drizzle of olive oil (if needed). If marinated, remove steak from marinade and discard marinade. Sear sliced steak for 2-3 minutes per side until cooked to desired doneness. Remove from pan and set aside to rest.
5. Sauté the Vegetables: In the same skillet used for steak, add sliced onion and bell pepper. Sauté for 5-7 minutes until softened and slightly browned.
6. Assemble and Serve: Slice rested steak against the grain into thin strips. Warm cauliflower tortillas if needed. On each tortilla, place some seasoned vegetables, top with steak strips, and add your favorite fajita toppings like guacamole, salsa, sour cream, and chopped cilantro. Enjoy!

Tips:

- Aim for medium-rare steak for the best texture and flavor.
- If you don't have a food processor, grate cauliflower florets using the coarse side of a box grater.
- Store leftover fajita fillings in an airtight container in the refrigerator for up to 3 days. Reheat gently in a pan or microwave.

Baked Cod with Asparagus and Hollandaise Sauce

Ingredients:

i. For the Baked Cod:

- 2 (4-6 oz) cod fillets
- 1 tablespoon olive oil
- Salt and freshly ground black pepper, to taste

ii. For the Asparagus:

- 1 pound asparagus, trimmed and ends removed
- 1 tablespoon olive oil
- Salt and freshly ground black pepper, to taste

iii. For the Low-Carb Hollandaise Sauce:

- 3 large egg yolks
- 1/4 cup unsalted butter, melted
- 1 tablespoon lemon juice
- Pinch of cayenne pepper (optional)
- Salt and freshly ground black pepper, to taste

Instructions:

1. Preheat the Oven: Preheat the oven to 400°F (200°C). Lightly grease a baking dish.

2. Prepare the Cod: Pat dry the cod fillets with paper towels. Season generously with salt and freshly ground black pepper. Place the seasoned fillets in the prepared baking dish and drizzle with olive oil.

3. Roast the Cod: Bake the cod for 10-12 minutes or until cooked through and flakes easily with a fork.

4. Prepare the Asparagus: While the cod is baking, toss the trimmed asparagus spears with olive oil, salt, and pepper.

5. Roast or Sauté the Asparagus:

  - Roasting: Spread the seasoned asparagus on a baking sheet and roast for 5-7 minutes alongside the cod until tender-crisp.
  - Sautéing: Heat a large skillet over medium heat, add the seasoned asparagus, and cook for 3-5 minutes until tender-crisp, turning occasionally.

6. Make the Low-Carb Hollandaise Sauce: In a blender or food processor, combine egg yolks, lemon juice, and a pinch of cayenne pepper. Blend until frothy. With the motor running, slowly drizzle in melted butter until the sauce thickens. Season with salt and pepper.

Tips:

  - Ensure not to overcook the cod to maintain its delicate texture.
  - If the hollandaise sauce is too thick, you can thin it out with warm water, adding a teaspoon at a time.
  - Leftovers can be refrigerated for up to 1 day, but the hollandaise sauce may separate. Reheat gently, whisking constantly.

Chicken Stir-Fry with Peppers, Onions, and Bok Choy

Ingredients:

i. For the Stir-Fry:

- 1 pound boneless, skinless chicken breasts or thighs, thinly sliced
- 1 tablespoon soy sauce (or coconut aminos for a gluten-free option)
- 1 tablespoon cornstarch (or arrowroot powder for a paleo option)
- 1 tablespoon vegetable oil
- 1 medium onion, sliced
- 1 bell pepper (red, yellow, or orange), sliced
- 1 head of bok choy, trimmed and separated into leaves
- 1 clove garlic, minced
- 1/2 cup chicken broth (or vegetable broth)
- 1 tablespoon rice vinegar (or white vinegar)
- 1 teaspoon sriracha (or your favorite chili sauce, optional)
- Salt and freshly ground black pepper, to taste

ii. Optional Garnish:

- Chopped green onions
- Sesame seeds

Instructions:

1. Marinate the Chicken: In a bowl, combine the sliced chicken with soy sauce and cornstarch. Allow it to marinate for 10-30 minutes.
2. Prepare the Vegetables: Slice the onion and bell pepper. Trim and separate the bok choy leaves. Mince the garlic.
3. Heat the Pan: Heat vegetable oil in a large wok or skillet over high heat.
4. Stir-Fry the Chicken: Add the marinated chicken to the hot pan and stir-fry until browned and cooked through. Set aside on a plate.
5. Sauté the Vegetables: In the same pan, sauté the sliced onion and bell pepper until softened and slightly browned.
6. Add Bok Choy and Garlic: Push the vegetables to one side of the pan and add bok choy leaves and minced garlic. Sauté until the bok choy starts to wilt.
7. Combine and Simmer: Pour in chicken broth, rice vinegar, and sriracha.

Bring to a simmer, scraping up any browned bits.

8. Return Chicken and Thicken (Optional): Add the cooked chicken back to the pan. If desired, thicken the sauce with a cornstarch slurry (1 tbsp cornstarch mixed with 2 tbsp water).

9. Season and Serve: Season the stir-fry with salt and pepper. Garnish with chopped green onions and sesame seeds if desired. Serve over cauliflower rice or low-carb noodles.

Tips:

- Ensure not to overcook the chicken to maintain its tenderness.
- Feel free to use other low-carb vegetables in place of bok choy.
- Adjust the level of spiciness by adding more or less sriracha.
- Leftovers can be stored and reheated for a quick meal later.

Stuffed Peppers with Ground Beef and Zucchini Noodles

Ingredients:

i. For the Stuffed Peppers:

- 4 bell peppers (red, yellow, orange, or a mix), halved and seeds removed
- 1 tablespoon olive oil
- 1 medium onion, chopped
- 2 cloves garlic, minced
- 1 pound ground beef (or ground turkey)
- 1 (14.5 oz) can diced tomatoes, undrained
- 1/2 cup chopped zucchini (optional)
- 1/2 cup chopped mushrooms (optional)
- 1 teaspoon chili powder
- 1/2 teaspoon dried oregano
- 1/4 teaspoon ground cumin
- Salt and freshly ground black pepper, to taste

- 1 cup shredded cheddar cheese (or your favorite cheese)

ii. For the Zucchini Noodles (Zoodles):

- 1 medium zucchini
- Spiralizer (or julienne peeler)
- 1 tablespoon olive oil (optional)
- Salt and freshly ground black pepper, to taste

Instructions:

1. Preheat the Oven: Set your oven to 375°F (190°C) and lightly grease a baking dish.
2. Prepare the Bell Peppers: Halve the bell peppers lengthwise, remove the seeds, and set them aside.
3. Optional Sautéing of Extra Vegetables: In a skillet over medium heat, sauté the onion in olive oil until softened. Add optional veggies like zucchini and mushrooms, and cook until tender.
4. Brown the Ground Beef: Add the ground beef to the skillet and cook until browned, breaking it up with a spoon as it cooks.
5. Simmer the Filling: Stir in the diced tomatoes, chili powder, oregano, cumin, salt, and pepper. Simmer for a few minutes until the flavors meld.
6. Prepare the Zucchini Noodles (Zoodles): Spiralize or julienne the zucchini into noodles.
7. Stuff the Peppers: Fill each bell pepper half with the ground beef mixture, then top with shredded cheese.
8. Optional Zoodle Bake: Toss the zucchini noodles with olive oil, salt, and pepper. Arrange them around the stuffed peppers in the baking dish.
9. Bake: Bake everything for 20-25 minutes until the peppers are tender and the cheese is melted and bubbly.
10. Serve: Enjoy your zesty stuffed peppers hot, accompanied by the baked zucchini noodles.

Tips:

- Pre-baking the peppers briefly can help ensure even cooking.
- Mix up the colors of the bell peppers for a visually appealing dish.
- Leftovers can be stored and reheated for convenient meals later on.

Variations:

- Add some red pepper flakes for extra spiciness.
- Garnish with fresh herbs like parsley or cilantro for added flavor.
- Swap out the ground beef for lentils or tempeh to make it vegetarian-friendly.

Shrimp and Cauliflower Rice Casserole

Ingredients:

For the Casserole:

- 1 head of cauliflower, riced (or 2 cups pre-riced cauliflower)
- 1 tablespoon olive oil
- 1 medium onion, chopped
- 2 cloves garlic, minced
- 1 pound shrimp, peeled and deveined (thawed if frozen)
- 1 (10 oz) can cream of mushroom soup (low-carb option)
- 1 cup milk (unsweetened almond milk or low-fat dairy milk)
- 1/2 cup shredded cheddar cheese
- 1/4 cup chopped fresh parsley
- 1 teaspoon dried thyme
- Salt and freshly ground black pepper, to taste
- 1/4 cup panko breadcrumbs (optional topping)

Instructions:

1. Preheat the Oven: Set your oven to 375°F (190°C) and lightly grease a baking dish.
2. Prepare the Cauliflower Rice: Use a food processor or box grater to rice the cauliflower. Alternatively, use pre-riced cauliflower.
3. Sauté the Vegetables: In a skillet over medium heat, sauté the onion in olive oil until softened. Add garlic and cook for another minute.
4. Cook the Shrimp: Season shrimp with salt and pepper, then cook in the skillet until pink and opaque. Remove and set aside.
5. Combine Cauliflower Rice and Creamy Sauce: In a bowl, mix cauliflower rice, cream of mushroom soup, milk, cheese, parsley, thyme, salt, and pepper.
6. Assemble the Casserole: Transfer the cauliflower mixture to the baking dish. Top with cooked shrimp.
7. Optional Panko Topping: Sprinkle panko breadcrumbs over the casserole for a crispy topping.
8. Bake: Bake for 20-25 minutes until bubbly and golden brown on top.
9. Serve: Spoon out and serve the delicious shrimp and cauliflower rice casserole.

Tips:

- Avoid overcooking the shrimp to keep them tender.
- Make a simple cream sauce if you don't have cream of mushroom soup.
- Store leftovers in the fridge for up to 3 days and reheat before serving.

Variations:

- Enhance with additional veggies like broccoli or mushrooms.
- Add red pepper flakes for a spicy twist.
- Roast the shrimp with herbs instead of sautéing for a different flavor profile.

Flank Steak with Chimichurri Sauce and Salad

Ingredients:

i. For the Flank Steak:

- 1 ½ pound flank steak
- 1 tablespoon olive oil
- Salt and freshly ground black pepper, to taste

ii. For the Chimichurri Sauce:

- ½ cup fresh parsley leaves, packed
- ¼ cup fresh cilantro leaves, packed
- 2 tablespoons olive oil
- 2 cloves garlic, minced
- 1 tablespoon red wine vinegar
- ½ teaspoon dried oregano
- ¼ teaspoon red pepper flakes (optional)
- Salt and freshly ground black pepper, to taste

iii. For the Salad:

- 4 cups mixed greens (romaine, arugula, or spinach)
- ½ cucumber, sliced
- ½ red onion, thinly sliced (optional)
- ¼ cup cherry tomatoes, halved (optional)
- 2 tablespoons olive oil
- 1 tablespoon lemon juice or balsamic vinegar
- Salt and freshly ground black pepper, to taste

Instructions:

1. Marinate the Steak (Optional): In a bowl, coat the flank steak with olive oil, salt, and pepper. Marinate for extra flavor.
2. Prepare the Chimichurri Sauce: Blend parsley, cilantro, olive oil, garlic, red wine vinegar, oregano, red pepper flakes, salt, and pepper until chunky. Alternatively, finely chop herbs for a rustic texture.
3. Make the Salad: Toss mixed greens, cucumber, red onion, and cherry tomatoes in a bowl.
4. Grill the Steak: Season the steak with salt and pepper, then grill for 4-5 minutes per side for medium-rare.
5. Assemble the Salad: Whisk olive oil, lemon juice (or balsamic vinegar), salt, and pepper for the dressing. Toss the salad in the dressing.
6. Rest and Slice the Steak: Let the steak rest for 5-10 minutes before slicing thinly against the grain.
7. Serve: Plate the salad and top with sliced steak. Drizzle chimichurri sauce over the steak or serve on the side.

Tips:

- Avoid overcooking flank steak to maintain tenderness.
- If grilling isn't an option, cook the steak in a hot skillet.
- Adjust red pepper flakes in chimichurri for desired spice.
- Include roasted vegetables for a complete meal.

Chicken Piccata with Zucchini Noodles

Ingredients:

i. For the Chicken Piccata:

- 2 boneless, skinless chicken breasts (4-6 oz each)
- ½ cup almond flour (or coconut flour)
- 1 tsp dried oregano
- ½ tsp garlic powder

- Salt and pepper, to taste
- 2 tbsp olive oil
- 2 tbsp butter
- ¼ cup dry white wine (or chicken broth)
- ¼ cup fresh lemon juice
- 2 tbsp capers, drained
- ¼ cup chopped fresh parsley (optional)

ii. For the Zucchini Noodles (Zoodles):

- 1 large zucchini (or 2 small zucchinis)
- Spiralizer (or julienne peeler)
- 1 tbsp olive oil (optional)
- Salt and pepper, to taste

Instructions:

1. Prepare Zoodles: Wash and spiralize zucchini into noodles.
2. Season Chicken: In a dish, mix almond flour, oregano, garlic powder, salt, and pepper. Dredge chicken in the mixture.
3. Cook Zoodles (Optional): Sauté zoodles in olive oil until tender-crisp, then set aside.
4. Cook Chicken: In a skillet, heat olive oil and butter. Cook chicken for 3-4 mins/side until golden and cooked through. Remove from pan.
5. Make Piccata Sauce: Deglaze the pan with wine, then add lemon juice and capers. Simmer until slightly thickened.
6. Finish and Serve: Return chicken to the pan, spoon sauce over it, and garnish with parsley. Serve with zoodles.

Tips:

- Ensure chicken is cooked to 165°F (74°C).
- Thin sauce with chicken broth if needed.

- Adjust capers to taste.
- Store leftovers in the fridge for up to 3 days.

Variations:

- Add minced garlic to sauce for extra flavor.
- Sprinkle red pepper flakes over zoodles for heat.

Eggplant Parmesan with Marinara Sauce

Ingredients:

i. For the Breaded Eggplant:

- 1 large eggplant (about 1 ½ pounds)
- ½ cup almond flour (or coconut flour)
- ¼ cup grated Parmesan cheese
- 1 tsp dried oregano
- ½ tsp garlic powder
- Salt and pepper, to taste
- 2 large eggs, beaten
- 2 tbsp olive oil

ii. For the Layered Casserole:

- 16 oz low-sugar marinara sauce
- 1 cup shredded mozzarella cheese
- ½ cup grated Parmesan cheese
- Fresh basil leaves, for garnish (optional)

Instructions:

1. Prepare Breading: In a shallow dish, combine almond flour, grated

Parmesan cheese, oregano, garlic powder, salt, and pepper.

2. Slice Eggplant: Cut eggplant into ½-inch thick rounds.

3. Bread Eggplant: Dip eggplant slices in beaten eggs, then coat with almond flour mixture.

4. Cook Eggplant: Heat olive oil in a skillet over medium heat. Cook breaded eggplant slices until golden brown and crispy. Drain excess oil.

5. Preheat Oven: Preheat oven to 375°F (190°C). Grease a baking dish.

6. Layer Casserole: Spread marinara sauce in the baking dish. Layer cooked eggplant slices, mozzarella, and Parmesan cheese. Repeat until ingredients are used, ending with cheese on top.

7. Bake: Bake for 20-25 minutes until cheese is melted and bubbly.

8. Serve: Garnish with fresh basil leaves and serve hot.

Tips:

- Salt eggplant slices to draw out moisture before breading.
- Substitute almond flour with panko breadcrumbs if desired.
- Store leftovers in the fridge for up to 3 days and reheat before serving.

Tofu Scramble with Vegetables and Avocado

Ingredients:

i. For the Tofu Scramble:

- 14 oz block firm tofu, drained and pressed
- 1 tbsp olive oil
- ½ medium onion, diced
- 1 clove garlic, minced
- ½ cup chopped mushrooms
- ½ cup chopped bell pepper (any color)
- ½ cup chopped broccoli florets (or other vegetables)
- ¼ cup nutritional yeast (or grated Parmesan cheese)

- 1 tsp turmeric powder
- ½ tsp smoked paprika
- Salt and pepper, to taste
- ¼ cup unsweetened almond milk (or water)

ii. For Serving:

- 1 ripe avocado, sliced
- Chopped fresh herbs (optional)
- Hot sauce (optional)

Instructions:

1. Prepare Tofu: Wrap tofu in a kitchen towel or paper towels and press with a heavy object for 15-20 minutes. Crumble tofu into scrambled egg-like pieces.
2. Sauté Vegetables: Heat olive oil in a skillet over medium heat. Cook onions until softened, then add garlic and cook for another minute. Add mushrooms, bell pepper, and broccoli, and cook until tender.
3. Season Tofu: Add crumbled tofu to the skillet. Stir in nutritional yeast, turmeric, smoked paprika, salt, and pepper. Pour in almond milk and cook for 3-4 minutes.

Serve and Enjoy:

- Divide tofu scramble among plates.
- Top with sliced avocado and fresh herbs.
- Add hot sauce for extra flavor if desired.
- Enjoy your protein-packed low-carb dinner!

6

Chapter 6

14-Day Carb Cycling Meal Plan for Women Over 50

This sample meal plan includes days with varying levels of carbohydrates, some high, some low, and some for resting, offering a well-rounded carb cycling strategy tailored for women aged 50 and over. You can modify serving sizes and food choices according to your personal taste and nutritional requirements.

Day 1 (High Carb):

- Breakfast: Greek Yogurt Parfait with Granola and Fruit
- Lunch: Lentil Soup with Whole-Grain Bread
- Dinner: Baked Chicken with Sweet Potato Mash and Green Beans

Day 2 (Low Carb):

- Breakfast: Eggs with Wilted Greens and Smoked Salmon
- Lunch: Chicken Caesar Salad
- Dinner: Salmon with Roasted Brussels Sprouts and Lemon Butter

Day 3 (High Carb):

- Breakfast: Whole-Wheat Pancakes with Nut Butter and Berries
- Lunch: Black Bean Burgers on Whole-Wheat Buns
- Dinner: Vegetarian Lasagna with Zucchini Noodles

Day 4 (Rest – Low Carb):

- Breakfast: Chia Pudding with Nut Butter and MCT Oil
- Lunch: Smoked Salmon Cream Cheese on Cucumber Slices
- Dinner: Flank Steak with Chimichurri Sauce and Salad

Day 5 (High Carb):

- Breakfast: Oatmeal with Nuts, Seeds, and Fruit
- Lunch: Quinoa Salad with Roasted Vegetables and Chickpeas
- Dinner: Teriyaki Salmon with Brown Rice and Edamame

Day 6 (Low Carb):

- Breakfast: Avocado Omelet with Cheese and Peppers
- Lunch: Grilled Shrimp with Zucchini Noodles and Pesto
- Dinner: Chicken Piccata with Zucchini Noodles

Day 7 (Rest – Low Carb):

- Breakfast: Hard-Boiled Eggs with Sliced Tomatoes and Avocado
- Lunch: Tuna Salad with Mixed Greens and Avocado
- Dinner: Eggplant Parmesan with Marinara Sauce

Day 8 (High Carb):

- Breakfast: Scrambled Eggs with Smoked Salmon and Whole-Wheat Toast

- Lunch: Turkey and Avocado Wrap on Whole-Wheat Tortilla
- Dinner: One-Pot Chicken and Veggie Paella

Day 9 (Low Carb):

- Breakfast: Protein Pancakes with Almond Flour and Berries
- Lunch: Taco Salad with Ground Beef, Lettuce Wraps, and Pico de Gallo
- Dinner: Shrimp and Cauliflower Rice Casserole

Day 10 (High Carb):

- Breakfast: Whole-Wheat French Toast with Berries and Maple Syrup
- Lunch: Creamy Tomato Pasta with Whole-Wheat Penne
- Dinner: Black Bean and Corn Quesadillas with Avocado Crema

Day 11 (Rest - Low Carb):

- Breakfast: Greek Yogurt with Chia Seeds and Berries
- Lunch: Ham and Swiss Roll-Ups with Mustard on Romaine Lettuce
- Dinner: Stuffed Peppers with Ground Beef and Zucchini Noodles

Day 12 (High Carb):

- Breakfast: Breakfast Burrito Bowl with Whole-Wheat Tortilla
- Lunch: Salmon with Brown Rice and Roasted Asparagus
- Dinner: Whole-Wheat Pasta Primavera with Seasonal Vegetables

Day 13 (Low Carb):

- Breakfast: Tofu Scramble with Vegetables and Avocado
- Lunch: Cobb Salad with Grilled Chicken, Avocado, and Blue Cheese
- Dinner: Steak Fajitas with Cauliflower Tortillas and Guacamole

Day 14 (Rest – Low Carb):

- Breakfast: Smoothie with Protein Powder, Greens, and Fruit
- Lunch: Soup and Salad (Split Pea Soup with Side Salad)
- Dinner: Baked Cod with Asparagus and Hollandaise Sauce.

7

Conclusion

Well done on taking the initiative to prioritize your health and delve into the realm of carb cycling! This journey towards purposeful nourishment has hopefully equipped you with delectable recipes and invaluable insights for a vibrant life beyond 50.

Keep in mind that carb cycling offers flexibility. Feel free to experiment with different meal plans to discover what suits your energy levels and lifestyle best. Along this journey, here are some key points to remember:

- Choose wholesome, unprocessed foods: Make fresh fruits, vegetables, whole grains, and lean proteins the cornerstone of your meals.
- Tune in to your body's signals: Notice how different carb levels affect your energy and adjust your plan accordingly to meet your hunger and energy needs.
- Embrace diversity: Explore a variety of recipes to keep your meals enjoyable and ensure you're receiving a wide array of nutrients.
- Celebrate your dedication: Consistency is key to the effectiveness of carb cycling.

This cookbook serves as a starting point. As you progress towards optimal health and well-being, always remember that YOU are the most essential ingredient. Embrace the transformative power of food to nourish your body and enrich your life. Happy cooking and happy carb cycling!